For permission requests, contact the publisher at:

HTA Books
High Touch Alliances
2634 Lakeforest Court
Dallas, Texas 75214
Phone: +1 (214) 803-9769

ISBN: 978-0-9822864-2-5 – $17.95
First Printing: February 2011
10 9 8 7 6 5 4 3 2 1

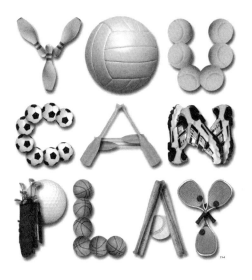

First Edition

• • •

Brenda Loube, M.S.

DEDICATION

    This book is dedicated to Fern Carness, who encouraged me to write a chapter in a book to tell my story. Fern Carness was a dear friend, colleague and one that mentored any woman who wanted her help. When she was in the beginning stages of planning her second edition of the "Wise Women Speaks" books, titled "Wise Women Speak: Choosing Stepping Stones Along the Path," she approached me to write a chapter in the book. I really had no desire to write a chapter and certainly not a book, but see what happens when someone believes in you! Fern has since passed from her battle with cancer. Her memories and gifts live on.

    Thanks Fern.

ACKNOWLEDGEMENTS

My life has been surrounded by so many teams: my family teams, work teams, sports teams, friendship teams, colleague teams, organizational teams, board teams, council teams, project teams, and my very own company team, Corporate Fitness Works.

In looking back, this has been an amazing journey these past five years. A student at one of my career development presentations at Towson University Exercise Science Class asked me what I was going to do next in my career. Without hesitation, I replied to her that I was going to write a book. Well, here is the book, so thank you to the student who asked the question.

I want to first thank my entire Corporate Fitness Works team for their support and giving me the opportunity to devote the time to write this book. A special thanks to Sheila for helping create the space I needed to write it.

To my sister Sharon, who has always been my biggest cheerleader and who has always been there for me. To Mom and Dad, I am so grateful for the support that you have given me throughout my life. I would like to personally honor my father for making play such an integral part of my life that I cherish play every day and carry on his family tradition. To my dearest friend Sarah, who has provided me daily support, for listening to me and helping to review and capture the essence of the book. To my brother, Jacky, who mentored me in ways I did not even know, especially athletically. Jacky was so instrumental in helping me develop my sports skills at a very young age. He taught me the fundamentals of many sports, particularly basketball and softball. Because of his innate coaching ability, I was able to excel in a number of sports. Thanks, Jacky, for all that you did to introduce me to and help me find my passion in sports. I would be remiss not to recognize your gift in helping me crystallize the final messages in my book.

I have an amazing family who has given me loads of fun while playing together. I want to thank my immediate family, Dad, Mom, Jacky, Debbie, Robyn, Richard, Sharon, David, Amanda and Mitchell for our wonderful annual beach vacations, playing whiffle ball, paddleball, and touch football games for the past 24 years and counting.

To all of my teammates from Montgomery Blair High School, Towson University, and the many fast-pitch softball teams that I played on, from the Plain Americans and the Virginians Team.

One of my coaches stood out. Sharma Wright, my high school coach at Montgomery Blair, volunteered her time to coach almost every sport at the time. Sharma encouraged me to pursue my athletic ability with fast pitch softball and I am forever indebted to her.

Mary Drohan, my business partner Sheila's mom, did not think twice about loaning us the money to start our business. Mary had the confidence and never looked back after she made such a huge financial commitment to both Sheila and me. She believed in us, and provided me with the experience of bringing health and fitness to Corporate America.

For over a year, Lisa Edwards helped to shape my original message and created the initial manuscript for the book. It was a lot of work but so much fun working with Lisa, who epitomized a teammate.

I also want to thank the over 2,000 participants who completed the Women and Team Play survey. Thanks for taking the time to complete this survey and for sharing the information that will help provide many invaluable statistics and ongoing stories to support the importance of women playing team sports.

I received over 400 requests from women to share their stories and I hope one day I will be able to showcase their stories on my web site. I would like to thank Sandy Slade, Fern Carness, Stephani Kolevar, Andrea Pent, Ellen Kandell, Dr. Jane Lynes, Cindy Sisson Hensley, Lyn St. James and Janet Tyler for taking the time to share your stories about how team sports impacted and changed your lives. Your stories wowed me.

I feel so blessed to have worked with Darlene Ellison and her publishing company, hta books, for believing in my message. Thanks for sharing your own experience and encouraging me along the way.

Thanks, Cynthia, for your coordination of the book. Lesley, thanks for doing a terrific job with the final editing and the flow of the book. Josh, you are one creative person who came up with an absolutely tremendous cover that matched my vision for a fun and unique display. Thanks, Brinley, for your creative brand for *You Can Play*.

I am so deeply grateful for all of you for helping me share the message to all women that *You Can Play*!

"On the basis of available participation research, the percentage of girls and women that annually participate in team sports is between 10% and 12% of the total population of females above age 6 in the United States."

William C. Beckner
Research Manager,
National Recreation and Park Association

FOREWORD

My passion is working with others to be the best they can be at what they do. For most of my life this has been WORK focused on people in business, in the business environment and on the skills necessary to be successful at business. WORK, WORK, WORK. It was not until my granddaughter began to participate in sports, and I began to coach girls' basketball, that I fully realized the extent to which positive experiences with sports, being a member of a team and the simple concept of PLAY had influenced me and, if conveyed appropriately, could influence others.

Around the same time, Brenda Loube approached me to discuss a book she was writing. Knowing my passion for collegiate sports and that I play recreational and USTA tennis, she knew I would be interested in its messages. She intended to focus on PLAY and the lessons learned from participating in team sports. What a great idea!

This book introduces us to PLAY or reminds us of the benefits of PLAY! Play? Repeat after me….PLAY! Sounds a lot different than WORK! Does the word PLAY make you smile? Does it scare you? Have you played since childhood? What if you never played organized sports? Is it possible to play again? Can PLAY and WORK mix? Do PLAY and WORK mix? Are there lessons from PLAY?

In my work and personal life, I have seen the benefits over and over again. At Pfizer, we experience the team model of "forming, storming, norming and performing," as all teams do. However, we strive to help our teams work quickly through the phases of the model in order to deliver a significant business goal – much like a basketball team coming together.

Another strong concept from the book is around decision-making and thinking on your feet. The business world continuously hits you with various scenarios and situations where critical thinking under pressure is required. In a game, a player is given the ball and must quickly evaluate the situation to make the best decision possible. This practice of decision-making on the court or field translates into quick thinking in the business world.

As a female leader, I've found that playing in sports has personally helped me to value the strengths of each person on my team and to be a better collaborator. In sports, you often have to adjust your game plan with changing situations and re-allocate resources to meet the goal of winning – key skills for succeeding in business. Everyone must play their part on a team and the team adjusts strategies as players rotate in and out – much like basketball. Encouragement and support helps each team member perform better and recover faster from mistakes.

Many of my mentees have played team sports and I often use sports stories and analogies to help them tackle challenges in their professions. For those who haven't played team sports, I encourage them to learn more about basketball or football so they can experience some of the examples of teamwork personally.

For many, PLAY reminds them of a time or of experiences that were extremely positive and in many cases shaped their very personality, style or level of self-confidence. Others hear the word PLAY and consider it something done only by kids. Still others consider it a silly notion and never relate the lessons learned from PLAY to their current success or to strengths or skills they may have today.

I wondered how I would feel when I read this book of lessons about PLAY. Growing up, I loved sports. Being close to Knoxville, Tenn. – the area was not only strong with men's collegiate sports but also with women's collegiate sports, thanks to Pat Summit and the University of Tennessee Lady Vols basketball team. Watching THE TEAM work together for success was clearly a concept I understood. Having a strong leader and strong support staff was also clearly understood. But there was a lot of raw talent there. Could lessons from sports translate to others even if they'd not played sports?

I decided to read the book with a fresh look and realized the direct influence that sports and play have had on me over time. I suspect you may have been impacted either positively or negatively through PLAY and sports in the same way that I have been. You may have a friend or loved one who gained confidence or became a better team member at work after becoming involved in PLAY.

Pick up this book and read the many lessons that Brenda and others have learned from their involvement in sports and PLAY experiences and if you aren't PLAYing today, now is the time! And remember........YOU CAN PLAY!

Pamela Prince-Eason is Vice President, Pfizer Worldwide Procurement. She also serves as Chairwoman of the Board for the Women's Business Enterprise National Council, as a Board of Trustees member of the Center for Strategic Sourcing Leadership and as a Global Committee Member for National Minority Supplier Development Council.

As a coach, a mentor and a grandmother, she encourages women and girls to participate in team sports and credits sports for helping her achieve success in business and in life.

TABLE OF CONTENTS

PROLOGUE:
WHAT IS YOUR
PLAY PERSONALITY?

Everyone has a play personality. Somewhere deep inside you lives a cheerleader, a coach, a star or a dedicated team member. When was the last time your play personality took over, allowing you to bask in the enjoyment of a game?

For too many of us, our play personality has been buried by a mound of work, family obligations, everyday responsibilities and the general whirlwind of life. We've lost the fun in life. Playtime has disappeared.

As a result, the only physical activities in which many women participate are of the "work" variety, such as cleaning, weeding the garden and performing other household maintenance. Some women exercise, but only in a regimented style devoid of enjoyment. In most cases, they exercise by necessity to lose weight or for health reasons as they age.

There is a big difference between exercise and play. The goal of this book is to help you experience both – at the same time. Suddenly, you will find yourself enjoying life more, getting healthy, and making lifelong friends who will support your health and fitness goals. I hope this book reminds you that once upon a time, you promised that you would play all the time when you were a grown-up.

But what if you're not a "natural" athlete? What if you have never set foot on a court or a field to play a team sport? Fortunately, it's never too late to play. Take it from someone who has made play a way of life.

A life grounded in play

I was raised in a household that valued team sports. As a result, sports have formed the fabric of my life. My father made everything a game that was both fun and challenging. Games were the center of family gatherings. At my paternal grandparents' house, the family spent hours playing step ball. When visiting my maternal grandparents, we joined our cousins in a game of touch football. Typically, I was one of the only girls to get in the game. How I dreaded the call from my parents that it was time to go in for dinner. Yet I always looked forward to the next opportunity to play.

My dad was a coach on the playing field and in life. Even today, he coaches my siblings and me whenever the opportunity presents itself. My father held high expectations and constantly challenged us to do better. There were times I wanted him to give more praise, to be more positive, or to say things I wanted to hear. But I have always appreciated that he took an interest, remained engaged and cared. Today, I realize there is not one "right" way to coach. In fact, home is an ideal place to try new things and learn about different team roles. This applies to both the coach and the player. At home, we are better able to handle constructive criticism, especially when it comes from a trusted family member. As my dad always said, anyone can tell you the good things you did. He helped me realize how I could improve, positioning myself for success. His passion was to help make the suggested improvements a reality and, as a result, help each of us win.

As a young girl, I loved growing and developing as an athlete. This included taking greater risks on a consistent basis. Beginning in elementary school, I could compete with the boys in my class as we played childhood games at recess.

I wanted to play baseball, but was told that I couldn't. After all, I was "only" a girl. In those days, girls did not have access to organized sports outside of school. I took advantage of all the school-sponsored high school sports teams that were available, including field hockey, softball, volleyball and basketball. When I reached high school, a coach recommended that I try out for a women's fast-pitch softball team. At the time, this was as close as women could get to professional sports. So at 16, I became the youngest player on the team.

In college, I continued to play on school teams – this time, softball and tennis. Then, in 1976, I was introduced to the sport where I would truly make my mark: racquetball. I became a nationally ranked player, ultimately winning several titles. In 1993, this led to my induction in the Jewish Sports Hall of Fame.

Sports also influenced and shaped my career. As a young woman, I earned a bachelor's degree in physical education and planned to be a P.E. teacher. Then, in the early 1980s, I became interested in health promotion and disease prevention. I wanted to prevent heart disease through early detection and education, and so began my journey to work in a preventative environment. At the time, I was working at a commercial health club as a program director. I had a vision for bringing fitness and health into the workplace. My business partner and I both quit our jobs, took the risk, and started Corporate Fitness Works, a company that designs and manages fitness centers for companies and retirement communities throughout the United States.

So can you play, too?

While I've always been interested in fitness, playing sports has shaped my life – including my personality, my confidence, my competitive spirit and my self-esteem. Play paved the way for me to achieve leadership roles as a high school and college coach, which then helped me better perform as a business owner.

What can play do for you? What do you need in your life today?

-   Shifting from "exercise" to "play" can have a profound impact on your health. Forget the quick fix of crash diets or horrendous exercise routines. Instead, focus on the enjoyment of moving and enjoying yourself through play. As a result, you will increase your physical activity level.

-   Team sports and other group physical activities can help you form new and long-lasting friendships with others who share similar goals.

- A play-focused life could provide enough physical activity to help prevent disease.

- Play offers an opportunity to release physical, mental and emotional stress.

The benefits are endless. All that is needed is a game plan. That's what you'll find on the following pages. You will find personal stories that will highlight the message in each chapter. At the close of each chapter, you will find a Playbook and a Workbook. In the Playbook section, you'll receive tips and reminders that can help you get the most from each chapter. For the Workbook section, I encourage you to put pen to paper and thoughtfully answer each question. Put in the time, and you will learn a great deal about yourself. Whether or not you have participated in team play in the past is unimportant, as you will soon come to realize that play is for everyone and *You Can Play*!

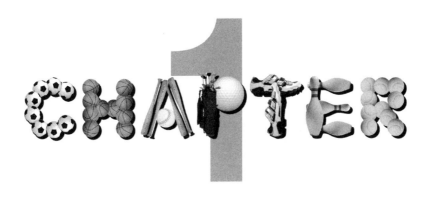

Life is a Playground

Picture yourself on the playground of life. Are you an active kid, enthusiastically trying out each piece of equipment, testing your limits and pushing yourself to the edge? Are you a quiet child, lolling on the swings and watching the others as they bond and play together? Or are you somewhere in between?

We can all remember times in childhood when we played with family members or friends. As adults, some look back on the playground with fondness, while others remember it with feelings of dislike and despair. We learned so many things from our experiences on the playground. Most of us never realized how much our time at play shaped the person we became. Yet today, these lessons affect our ability to succeed – in play and in life.

After all, shouldn't adult life be a playground where we actively stretch our minds and bodies and have fun doing it? For some of us, though, our view of play was molded and shaped through less-than-ideal childhood experiences. Understanding the impact of those "playground" events on your life can help you unlock a new world of play and enjoyment. And it all starts on the seesaw.

Lessons from a playground

Every child has a favorite area of the playground. Some like the swings and the seesaw, while others are drawn toward the merry-go-round or the monkey bars. Watch a child at the playground over time, and you will see her advance through phases with each activity. She will try something new, play it as often as she can, improve, and share her excitement as she masters the game.

Just as they will throughout life, children tend to gravitate toward activities where they perform well, enjoy themselves and find companions. The seesaw, for instance, is one of the best examples of early team play. It requires that partners work together. So if a child wants to play on the seesaw, she must ask someone else to play with her. As you know, without a partner the seesaw does not work. The team must plan and adjust based on who is heavier and who is lighter. The pair must work together physically. Only when these steps are followed can play become fun and successful. Throughout the process of playing on the seesaw, team members discover that their choice of playmates has a direct impact on their experience. Do you see the life lessons being revealed through play?

In fact, your specific childhood experiences during play with others shaped your perspectives, patterns and behaviors throughout your life. For instance, during recess or P.E. class, you probably had the option of playing kickball or dodgeball. A majority of children – especially girls – preferred kickball over dodgeball for several reasons. Dodgeball required more agility and skill, as well as generating moments of fear and intensity. Let's face it, not many girls wanted to run the risk of getting smacked in the head with a ball. The goal was to publicly hit other players and, if successful, take them out of the game. It was a contest of elimination rather than inclusion. Girls would stand behind the boys, looking for protection. In doing so, young girls were taught that the role of a braver team member was to take the risk and shield them from the challenge, allowing them to hide to avoid the issues and responsibilities of getting in the game.

Kickball, on the other hand, offered an atmosphere of inclusion. Just about anyone, boy or girl, could play successfully by kicking a large ball, running the bases, and attempting to catch or stop the ball. Everyone was able to enjoy the team atmosphere of playing with others.

Consider your childhood playground experience. Was it filled with positive kickball moments, where you felt a part of a team? Was it peppered with dodge ball excitement, where you were thrilled by competitive drive? Or was it plagued by fear and unhappiness, where you tried to hide from potential embarrassment or pain? How have those experiences and feelings affected your view of play in your life today?

"You can't play"

Play is inherently good. That's one reason children are instinctively drawn to it. Yet each child's approach to play is affected by her innate personality. For example, some children are high achievers in whatever they do, attacking each new game as a challenge to be conquered. Others are natural athletes who can perform well in any sport. These two groups, however, make up a relatively small portion of the population. For everyone else, group play is more likely to be successful when it is encouraged.

Unfortunately, many children experience the exact opposite. They enjoy playing and being part of the group – until someone tells them they cannot. A child is picked last for the team. Classmates laugh when a child trips, drops a ball or runs more slowly than the others. A parent implies that a child isn't strong enough, coordinated enough or good enough to try out for the team.

As a child, I always wanted to play baseball. I was a quiet and shy young girl when I was told that I couldn't play, as only boys played baseball. My competitive personality saw this as a challenge, which led to a lifelong love and enjoyment of softball. But what about other girls and women, who didn't have the family encouragement and mentorship I enjoyed? Do they – even now, perhaps decades later – still believe they can't play or whether or not play can be an integral part of their life?

Act like a lady

This leads to another cultural factor that particularly affects women. In the United States, as in much of the world, competition among women is not always considered acceptable. Women with a drive to win and succeed garner negative comments, while their male counterparts are lauded for these same qualities. Why? Perhaps because women are, by nature, givers. Historically, women have been praised for other accomplishments that are appropriately classified as supporting roles.

Unfortunately, these attitudes and perceptions lead many women away from participating on sports teams, and discourage them from wanting to compete and win. It takes practice and drive to maintain a competitive spirit and be successful. To accomplish this, women must work with – not against – their natures. For example, competing to win and supporting others can go hand-in-hand. It is possible to do your personal best, play fair and rise to the top gracefully.

Sports does not take away a woman's femininity, nor does it imply that she has masculine tendencies. A woman can be competitive, hard-driving and determined in a sport, or she can just sit back, relax and play. In either case, she's still a woman who should not let cultural stereotypes define her or inhibit her from joining a team.

Running the rat race

Today, play is not something that naturally fills children's free time. It is not the activity they look forward to after school and on weekends. Instead, children now see play as a chore that their mother enforces by turning off the television, computer or video game. Play is scheduled between layers of responsibilities and organized activities that parents feel are important to raising a child in today's competitive world.

The same holds true for adults. In Corporate America, we are highly disciplined and scheduled to the hilt. There is no siesta each day to revive ourselves. We don't give ourselves permission to take a long holiday as in Europe, where they shut down to relax for a month.

I recently met a woman with a simple solution that many may see as radical. A dedicated racquetball player, she modifies her work schedule so that she can keep a standing time on the court each week. Unfortunately, most adults don't view play as important or productive. As a result, they don't prioritize the time to exercise or take care of themselves as they should. I am here to tell you, playing will transform your life. Once you add some form of play into your schedule, your life will change in positive ways you can't imagine.

Make play a priority – today

When recalling your own childhood experiences, consider how this experience has changed for kids today. Play has dramatically changed, in very unfortunate ways, for children today. Those changes could be doing damage to your own children or grandchildren. Children have no idea what they are missing.

The lack of true play is an absolute shame. Kids are missing out on an incredible opportunity to experience invaluable life events. You can't turn back the clock for children who have been brought up in a culture that minimizes playtime. But you can help kids reap the rewards of play moving forward. In other words, it is never too late to create the opportunity for new and different experiences through play.

How do we regain the value of playing outside after school rather than sitting in front of the computer screen playing video games? Do we need to build more indoor playgrounds to change how kids think about play? Do we need to accommodate more safety concerns so parents will allow more play? Or is it simply that we as adults need to truly see the value of play in our own lives in addition to the lives of our children?

We certainly need to evaluate the institutions that influence our children. Recess has been cut out of the school day for a variety of reasons: possible lawsuits, sale of playground space to ease budget concerns, and more time for academic development. But to develop the whole person, children need to play, run, have fun, and learn the personal skills and life lessons that come along with this interaction. When children run free and play, they build a variety of life skills that include sharing, self-confidence and contributing to a team.

Unless you get in the game and play, you have no idea what you are missing. Too many women who were discouraged from playing as children have never had the experience of being on a sports team. They have no idea what their children and grandchildren may end up missing as well.

As a future mother, or grandmother, you can move beyond your childhood fears and experiences to get in the game – today. This might mean slowly reintroducing the idea of play, at your own pace. For example, get on that bike that sits idle in the garage and ride around the block. Perhaps this simple step will remind you how much play can add to your life.

This can lead to another exciting experience – playing on a team for the first time. Then, it will be easier to expose your own daughter or granddaughter to team sports, with a chance to try out everything from soccer, T-ball, volleyball and softball to basketball, racquetball, tennis and more.

Why do this, you say? Play enhances your physical and mental health. It can also boost success in your adult roles as a business partner, parent, family member, volunteer or professional. Best of all, "play" is synonymous with "fun"! If you can be better, feel better and have more fun, why let the children keep all the playing for themselves?

Sweep away the negative experiences of childhood. Don't allow fears and other barriers to stop you from making play a priority in your life. Instead, focus on the positive or important aspects of play. If you are not playing currently, give yourself permission to play. Ask yourself why you are not playing with your child, your significant other and your neighbors. What makes you feel like you don't deserve to play? Were there experiences in your past that keep you from wanting to play on a team?

You can play in any arena you choose. The ball is in your court and, if you want to pick up the ball and play, you can!

Playbook
As you consider getting into the game, keep these tips in mind:

1. ## Make play one of your top five priorities.
   If you've never had a great experience playing on a team, you probably omitted team play from your to-do list as an adult. Guess what? It's time to rewrite your to-do list! Play down your feelings that you will fail, and play up the opportunity for a new experience in your adult life. You never know what you are missing until you have tried. I challenge you to play something new and different that you have always wanted to try. Start a neighborhood volleyball game one night a week or sign up for a recreational soccer league. If there were a whiffle ball or kickball league, would you play? The experience ahead of you is so amazing that you will ask yourself, "Why have I been waiting so long to sign up and play?"

Business Owner Spins Basketballs Into Gold

As long as I can remember, I have been physically active. I was a member of a variety of sports teams as a child. In high school and college, I played golf, tennis, softball, volleyball and basketball.

I look back fondly on my experience playing Division I college basketball, when the demands left little time for anything other than basketball and school. I did not take for granted that I was one of the first women to reap the rewards of Title IX, with a full ride to play ball.

As a young adult, I can remember wondering if all the effort was worth being a part of that Division I team. Ultimately, my answer was always, "Yes!" Looking back on my college basketball experience now, I firmly believe that I learned more about life through teamwork on that court than I ever did in the classroom.

This experience also helped me create a niche as an entertainer and develop a childhood dream into a million-dollar business. At 12 years old, I watched a lady put on a performance spinning and dribbling basketballs. Her act left such an impression on me that, even then, I knew I was going to spin basketballs for a living. For 22 years, I entertained at schools, camps, NBA and WNBA games, and college halftimes, as well as special events throughout the world. It was a wonderful way to make a living.

On reflection, being part of a team taught me how to be successful in my life, even after my ability to play at a competitive level was limited. Being a business owner is not for wimps. I compare it to the intensity of playing in a game. No doubt, my ability to build and work with my team made all the difference. I learned to handle adversity, the value of dedication and sacrifice for long-term success, the rewards of working as a team, and how to work well with others. I learned that persistence and dedication pay off, that you have to sacrifice things initially in order to achieve long-term success for the common goal, and that winning and losing is a part of life. These lessons have become part of the fabric of who I am today.

Sandy "Spin" Slade
Former Professional Basketball Entertainer,
Entrepreneur, Creator and Founder of Skillastics®

2.   **Overcome your barriers.**

The only thing stopping you is – you. Is the fear of the unknown standing in your way? You just need a simple strategy to break down your barriers:

- Turn loose any negative experiences from the past.

- Set your mind on building new, positive experiences.

- Identify a sport or activity that you know you will enjoy and can be successful in trying. Just try it.

- Find others who will encourage you to try something new. Make a commitment to enjoy the experience together.

- If you are unable to find something that fits your interests, start something yourself. Invite others to join you in your game, right where you need it to be. I guarantee there are others out there who have the same game in mind, but are too afraid to extend the invitation themselves.

3.   **Let play evolve to fit your life changes, and always play with others.**

Play not only looks different for each of us as individuals, but our definition of play will also evolve and change during our lifetime. We may move from competitive, high-intensity sports to versions of play more realistic for our age and interests. Thank goodness for retirement communities which offer sports and opportunities for play such as golf, tennis, pool, bridge, swimming, bocce ball, poker and even active video games for playtime. There is nothing better than seeing a group of friends playing their way through retirement. Chances are, these same people played their way through their careers as well.

For me, play is a way to relax, unwind and let go of stress in my life. I look forward to any type of competitive play. Each person needs to define play for herself. Whatever it looks like to you, play each day and enjoy it!

Workbook
To assess your commitment to play, ask yourself these questions:

1. As a child, what did you enjoy most about playing?

2. If play is not a part of your life today, what are you missing?

3. What do you hope to gain from incorporating play into your life?

4. What is your greatest fear concerning team sports?

5. What strategy will help you overcome that fear?

6. Who in your life can cheer you on, tag along for the experience and help keep you motivated?

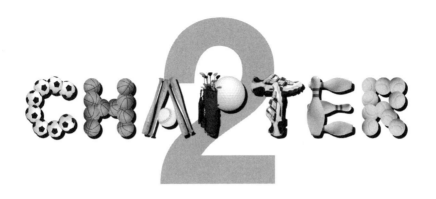

Life Takes Teamwork

People perform better when working as a team. This might mean a family, a circle of friends, a work team or the community. And the team might have a membership of two or 2,000.

You first learned about teamwork as a young child within your own unique family. This experience taught you about the positive – and the not-so-positive – aspects of teamwork. For better or worse, you don't get to choose your immediate family members. Family, however, provided the original team concept and environment where you learned to be yourself and develop the necessary skills to succeed on future teams.

Family was always there watching: your first step, your first day at school and your first move away from home. Your family helped you take risks and get outside of your comfort zone, and pushed you to be your best. They were in prime position to be your best supporters and fans when time to celebrate your victories.

Consider a baby's first steps. Children are endlessly coached and encouraged to walk. When the baby at last succeeds in taking those few, tentative steps, mom and dad spread the good news far and wide. This ritual of encouragement and celebration repeats itself at other milestones, like the first new tooth and the first day of school. But then, children grow up. They enter high school and college. As young adults, they launch their chosen careers. They lose the perspective and the value placed on milestones and first steps. In addition, adolescents entering adulthood often develop a fear – starting during the teen years – of being vulnerable to their family "team" and revealing their hopes, dreams and plans for the future. One of the benefits of being on a team is that it provides a safe environment in which to take risks. As this teen/adult child constructs a wall to barricade herself from her family team, the benefits stop running. The encouragement, celebration and coaching might even disappear. But will the lessons gained from the teamwork during adolescence remain for a lifetime? How can families keep that teamwork alive?

Balancing the good with the bad

The key to gaining the benefits of a team is openness. When you take the risk of exposing your thoughts, dreams and ideas to the team (or in this case, the family), you give others a chance to help you be your best. The foundation for this confidence was established when your parents, siblings and extended family played the role of coach or fellow teammate during childhood. If they accepted you, allowed you to make mistakes and redirected you in a positive way, you continued to try until you eventually succeeded.

Of course, family members and other team members you deal with early in life are not perfect. Sometimes, our family and young friends fall short of our expectations for being the perfect team members and, to some extent, this knowledge teaches us teamwork. It also teaches us to find the positive in another's approach even if it's a different style than we would choose. Teamwork is about building relationships, and relationships help shape our life experiences.

This is repeated with other teams throughout our lifetime – at school, at work and at play. Team relationships teach us about ourselves, help us develop new skills and push us to succeed. Some team members serve as mentors or coaches. Others function as a sounding board. One team member may be someone you watch and learn from, but of whom you don't ask questions. Some team members will usurp the role you wished to play on the team; others may encourage you to play differently than they do.

A strong team can be defined in so many different ways. A successful and productive team is better for the diversity in styles, personalities, interests, talents, strengths and approaches of its members. It is the complexity of a team that makes it strong – because it is multi-faceted and because of the work that must be done to bring diverse people together to reach a common goal.

When my business partner and I first launched our company, we didn't realize how different we were as individuals. Fortunately, those differences resulted in a combination that made a strong team. In turn, we developed a strong, complementary team within our company. We learned that if everyone was the same, the team would have so many challenges that it would be difficult to accomplish our goals. By bringing our unique capabilities to the team, and then respecting and trusting those differences, we were able to build on each others' strengths. That was one of the keys to our success.

A training ground for life

Teamwork is increasingly important in life. The ability to form relationships and build team concepts is considered key to corporate success, yet at the same time, technology is taking the place of face-time. Many team members embrace the ease and speed of communicating by e-mail, or voice mail or texting, which precludes them from learning interpersonal skills and other basics of teamwork.

In Chapter 1, we explored why play is critical. We now know that teamwork is a valuable skill in any aspect of life. But to become the consummate team member – in any setting – you must combine the two. Playing on a team is the central ingredient to making the most of the teamwork experience. Our ability to form relationships and build teams affects all aspects of our lives, and working well on a team is an acquired behavior. Consider the following questions as they relate to your everyday teamwork experiences:

- How do you contribute to the team?

- Are you taking advantage of your opportunities to create relationships?

- Is your team working together as a well-oiled machine?

The ability to function as a member of a team is fundamentally valued, whether we are playing roles in the workplace on project teams, in our communities, as volunteers, as members of a book club or quilting circle, or as a friend or family member. On some level, team-like experiences present themselves in virtually every dimension of our lives. Our best opportunity to learn to be a great team member is in play, where we can learn from our mistakes in an atmosphere where our passion and thrill for the game run strong.

When we play for fun, while valuing the team approach, we create the most successful outcome. Team players put themselves in their teammates' shoes: fix mistakes and move on to the next play. Each day, there are a million opportunities to approach life with these shared values and ethics.

Playing with others on a team is a training ground for life. If you are a parent, you have applied this knowledge with your own children. Play dates, play groups and playtime are expected facets of childhood development. There are even play dates for moms, who in watching their children's play behavior, have come to recognize that play is good for them as well.

As time progresses, team play grows more complex as expectations and demands of family and work grow more stressful and demanding. We need to get back to basics so that we can have fun and just play. We can never return to sharing a toy at the age of two, but we do need to rise to these new tough challenges of budgets and relationships. The concepts of play and team, and the lessons associated with each, provide an excellent transition for learning from child to adult.

Making choices

As a child, you most likely decided to join a team based on peer pressure, common interests, skills or perceived goals. But during adulthood, the possibilities for growth change things dramatically. You may choose a team because of its members' differences rather than their similarities.

If you are open to meeting others in their comfort zones, extending your own as a result, you can learn new things. Only you can choose to take the risk and associate with those who will build you up and help you expand your skills and experience. Rather than choosing a team of individuals just like you, you may join a team where you can learn to value, respect and trust others who are different.

A group of women had been playing racquetball together for many years, and they invited me to join their group on a regular basis. The game was not new to me, but the dynamics of the group made this both a risk and an opportunity to grow and learn. As a result of stepping out of my comfort zone, I had an absolute blast. As is expected when a new team member joins an existing team, I had a long way to go to understand and appreciate the intricacies of the individuals and the team they had built.

As women, we are good at putting the puzzle together, determining who others are and how we fit into the picture. We are the matchmakers for our friends and family, yet we sometimes forget to make appropriate matches for ourselves! This tendency for women to coordinate a group and bring people together creates a distinct advantage in team building and an opportunity to become a valued member of a team. We can contribute, appreciate others who contribute, and understand how we complement each other. Our challenge, however, is to take these inherent skills to the playing field. Whether playing as a young girl or an adult, there are many skills to be learned through the experience. Two very important core skills are adaptation to change and relationship-building.

Teams are dynamic. Membership changes, the leagues that teams play in change and players on a team try out new roles. Nothing stays the same. While this may seem like a challenge, in fact it helps us as individuals. We learn to adapt and thrive under a variety of circumstances.

After all, as we move through life, the teams we establish and get comfortable with are bound to change. By introducing new members, we shift team dynamics – sometimes not as we would like, but always for the betterment of having had the experience. The quick and constant changes on teams help us acclimate to change in the groups we will belong to later in life. If there is an injury or if we are rotating in and out of play, the dynamics of the team will change many times over the course of a single game.

Have you ever heard of the expected team-building experience of forming, storming, norming and performing? It refers to the necessary steps of coming together; working through the discomfort of new roles, strengths and weaknesses; getting to know one another and becoming comfortable; and then really getting it right. Completing these steps can take years, or it can take a matter of minutes. For those of us who have practiced and played on teams, the process occurs without much mental, emotional or physical energy. For those of us without the experience in team play, the process can be overwhelming and somewhat debilitating.

When we are deciding which team to join or become acquainted with, we tend to lead with the things that make us most comfortable. This familiar role, whatever it might be, will inevitably change over the course of your life. In fact, your role may change over the course of the day. You may be a grandmother, mother, aunt, daughter, spouse, life partner, co-worker, business owner, executive, manager, assistant, leader, coach and team member during different times in your life – or all at the same time. Regardless of your role, you will find that in each situation, common bonds will bind your team. Additionally, there is something to be said about the emotional bond and the hook that keeps people going back for more of the same team experience. Common bonds in team play make the activity more inviting and enjoyable and a platform to have fun. Just as every person eats and sleeps, everyone wants to play and have fun. It is inevitable that we adapt to change.

The well-rounded team member

Practice makes perfect. And in terms of teamwork, playing with a sports team is a great way of practicing your overall relationship skills.

In general, we don't practice at relationships. We just forge ahead and expect to get it right.

When done well, teamwork looks easy. As a result, we think we should instinctively know how to be an effective team member. After all, we forge ahead in our families, work teams and busy lives, even if a particular interaction or relationship isn't going well.

But when a team does not perform well, the situation drains our mental and physical energy. It becomes twice as hard to accomplish goals. Frustration and other negative emotions rob us of our energy and our time. The situation divides camps. Walls are constructed that, once detected, are not easily brought down. In other words, a dysfunctional team can be a life-changing experience, too. The stress can threaten our physical health, while also robbing us of the gratifying feelings that accompany team success.

With so much at stake in our everyday lives and pursuit of happiness, wouldn't it be most prudent to practice our relationship and teamwork skills in a non-threatening environment? Sports teams provide that environment, where working toward a common goal and fitting in with others is rewarding.

When you play on a team, not only do you learn to adapt, change and build relationships, but you also learn to empathize, sympathize, and consider the needs, unique value and strengths of others. Being a team member can build self-esteem. It helps you uncover and come to understand your own strengths, as well as how you can complement others. We've all seen the difference a self-confident woman can make in a board room, PTA meeting or work group.

Teamwork is the backbone of working well with others, whether your team is on a court, field, conference room or in your kitchen. It requires the ability to appreciate a range of personalities, playing styles and work ethics to form a cohesive group. On successful teams, all members work together toward a common goal, create a shared work ethic, keep an outcome-oriented spirit, and share the responsibility to succeed. Coaches teach team members by rewarding and complimenting them for their contributions to the success of the team, not just their ability to score individually. More importantly, great coaches recognize team members' efforts to go beyond previous contributions by taking risks, thus maximizing their potential. Leaders encourage their team members to push and achieve to do their best and to consistently raise the bar.

Being a team is about working together, learning about each other, seeking to appreciate each other, and then learning to succeed together. Delivering on common goals is one of the greatest highs you can experience. It comes from knowing that if you work hard together and appreciate the way you complement each other, you can exceed your collective expectations as a team. Best of all, this principle can be practiced on the field or the court, and then applied to every team in your life.

Breast Cancer Survivor Leaves Comfort Zone to Race Dragon Boats

I've exercised throughout my life and was an aerobics instructor years ago, but team sports were not valued or emphasized in my childhood home. It was not until I was married and my children were grown that I got out of my comfort zone. At about age 40, I joined a dragon boat racing team made up of breast cancer survivors. The experience changed my life.

When I arrived at the first meeting to sign up, I was more interested in what I should wear than how I should row. In fact, I spent so much time chatting with the others, I forgot to add my name to the list of interested participants. As a result, I landed on the alternate team. In the beginning, I had to be on the sidelines waiting for a space to open in the boat. But wait I did.

I never could have imagined how much work it takes to get 20 women to paddle in a completely synchronized fashion for three minutes! It looks effortless when it's done right. But to make it seem so easy, the team has been on the river early in the morning, day after day, feeling cold, tired and even sick.

Being on this team has taught me about cooperation and compromise: pushing myself to work with others for a common goal, hitting the water with each paddle at precisely the same instant. The team showed me that winning is possible, if everyone gives it all they've got. And what an amazing experience that common success can be! I apply these insights daily in my interactions with my husband, children, grandchildren, business partners and customers.

Fern Carness
MPH, RN, Entrepreneur

Playbook
As you focus on your teamwork skills, keep these tips in mind:

1. **Evaluate your skills.**
   Think about the skills you bring to a team. Whether you are a spectator, supporter, player, captain or coach, you can impact others in a positive way.

2. **Remember that teamwork takes practice.**
   Just like any other skill, it takes practice and dedication to become a successful team member. Work on soft skills such as reflective listening, openness to new ideas, strong work ethic and dedication. These will pay enormous dividends over time.

3. **Recognize your own successes.**
   Find the confidence it takes to step out in an attempt to influence others.

Workbook
Reflect for a moment and ask yourself these questions:

1. How can you take personal risks that will make you a better team member?

2. Are there teamwork skills you have developed at work that could apply on the field, or vice versa?

3. What are two actions you could take today that would improve your participation as a team member?

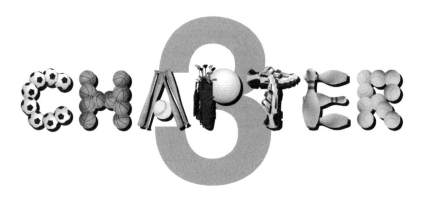

Soaring Above Your
Own Expectations

What if the key to your success depended on being a member of a team?

This may sound like a strange formula for self-improvement, but working as part of a team can assist a woman to reach performance levels she never thought possible. It all starts with accepting new challenges and trying new approaches, then quickly moving to accomplish major goals and reach milestones that may have once seemed impossible.

Of course, trying new techniques and testing new environments are notions that come naturally to children. If you had the opportunity to play on a team during childhood, you probably moved around and played various positions. Don't underestimate the impact this experience had on your overall development. This important phase of growing up should be seized whenever possible. If, however, you missed the opportunity to experience this level of team play as a child, you can still get in the game as an adult first-timer. It's never too late to try it out for yourself.

Yet too often, older children and adults are forced to specialize in one area and don't get to try new stuff. Consider my situation growing up playing on a softball team. I played second base. I knew the position well and could handle all of its ins and outs. On my team, I was considered the second-base expert, and the team wanted me to take ownership of that position. What's more, my teammates expected me to play second base at the highest possible level of skill and to execute with minimal mental mistakes and errors. Luckily for me, I enjoyed playing that role, specializing in all aspects of perfecting the position of a second baseman.

Why do individuals end up specializing in specific roles? Most often, it is as a result of utilizing team members' strengths. The third baseman needs great reflexes and reaction skills. The shortstop must be quick and able to cover a lot of ground and have a strong arm.

While this specialization is understandable and even desirable in highly competitive arenas, it can be a trap as well because it limits opportunities to try new things. Adults who may not have experienced team play when younger are already faced with a challenge to simply find the right activity and get into the game. Don't allow yourself to be limited by what others see as your strengths. Try new things that you may be interested in doing. Better still, seek out a team that will support you in developing skills in your areas of interest – not in areas where you are most naturally gifted.

Pushing beyond your limits

Chances are, you are painfully aware of your limitations. But are you aware that it's easier to push beyond those limitations when you're part of a team?

Everyone has strengths that we are drawn to as well as weaknesses in areas we tend to shy away from. Individually, it is easier to excel in the dimensions of life where you are naturally gifted. But by yourself, it can be difficult to develop and grow in areas where you've always had challenges. If you take on more difficult personal challenges and succeed, you may experience the unequaled thrill of satisfaction.

Team play is an incredible tool for this kind of growth. In team play, you are exposed to situations where others are there to help, assist and boost your morale. Team members frequently provide the needed encouragement and motivation to achieve success – success you may not have achieved on your own. Some team members have strengths that mirror your own, while others offer a completely different skill set. This creates opportunities to learn from one another and push each other to go further.

Playing on a team also provides a setting to try activities you might not otherwise have attempted for fear of failure. Your team members have a vested interest in advising and supporting you, as well as tying up loose ends, especially in areas of uncertainty and limited experience. If you are flying solo, you are limited to activities you can accomplish by yourself. On a team, you can stretch beyond these limits, thanks to team members who can back you up and catch you when you fall.

Special challenges women face

Pushing beyond limits does not come easily, especially for women. A number of factors attract women to work only in a team setting, rather than pushing to achieve as individuals. These factors include an overall history of nurturing, a dearth of role models, low levels of self-confidence, and a general aversion to risk-taking.

This behavior, however, is not a healthy one as an individual. Traditions, for the most part, still influence roles we each play, whether in the home, workplace or community. For example, it is still uncommon to find a man who stays at home to take control of domestic duties, permitting his spouse the ability to focus her emotional and mental energy on her career. Traditionally, women have a unique role in strengthening the family unit. This role does not encourage a woman's individual growth and development, but rather provides the stability that allows other family members to develop and pursue their interests. When the most basic needs of home, family and health are met, it's much easier to take risks in other areas of life.

For instance, when I was a child, my mother managed our household. She made certain that my siblings and I were free to challenge ourselves in all areas of development. I always intended to go to college and earn an undergraduate degree. But, as I advanced through my educational journey, I became intrigued with cardiac rehabilitation. No one encouraged me to pursue this field or to earn a graduate degree. Yet throughout college, my involvement in team sports sparked the ambition and drive, and I went on to graduate school.

Women also face evolving roles in the workplace, while still stuck in some of the paradigms of generations past. While male counterparts typically enjoy recognition, women tend to shy away from accolades and instead forge ahead to the next task. This approach makes it more difficult for women to step out and exceed expectations.

Perceptions of men and women also remain different in the workplace.

For example, when a man takes a business risk that does not turn out as anticipated, it is generally viewed for what it is: a learning experience. In contrast, when a woman takes a risk and it does not turn out as planned, it is often viewed in terms of her inferior ability. The long-standing perception of gender differences in the workplace is slowly dissipating. But for those of us who have worked in this culture, playing it safe is often the preferred choice for women.

In addition, women are trained to see self-improvement and challenges differently than most men. This extends to every aspect of life, including sports. In softball, for example, each team sets a batting order based on individual success rates. Most women are content just to be in the game. We won't push to move up to bat higher in the order. Instead, we tend to settle in and grow content. If a woman is the No. 6 batter, she assumes that the team needs her in that spot and she'll stay there.

Saying goodbye to limits – everywhere

Pushing beyond your limits applies to all areas of life. For example, there is a strong link between extending beyond your comfort zone and increasing your self-confidence. Confidence comes from challenging yourself and reaching for success. The improved confidence, together with positive reinforcement once success is achieved, will ultimately free you to extend your limits.

This is where the experience of team play is so valuable. Being a member of a team motivates you and gives you the confidence to push yourself beyond your defined limits. It's the perfect place to begin building self-confidence. After all, isn't it less risky to push yourself and exceed expectations in play, rather than in the professional arena?

As an example, imagine your job requires you to manage money entrusted to you by an organization. It's expected that you will garner an acceptable rate of return on investment. Or, if you lead a team of volunteers raising funds for a worthy cause, you are responsible for accomplishing a very specific goal. In these examples, where interests of others are involved, your level of flexibility is extremely small. Taking risks would not be responsible.

But let's say you have just joined a beginners' volleyball league and are learning the game. Initially your position is likely to just strike the ball and keep it in the air for a teammate. As you strengthen your game, you may be the one to send the ball back over the net. But if you fail to strike the ball, the game is not lost. It may not even mean a point for the other team. There are many more points to be made, and the outcome of the game does not affect your income or your career. If you make a mistake in play, you can simply move on with the intention of doing better next time. You must buy into this philosophy!

This experience builds character in so many ways. Even when you serve, whether or not the ball makes it over the net does not end the game. Rather, it is just a part of the larger picture. Later, you will rotate into the server's position again with more experience under your belt. You will have more chances to serve. You will touch the ball many times in a game. The more you touch the ball, the more you will contribute to getting it over the net, and the more you will succeed.

Yes there is a risk every time you step on the court to play – there is a risk your team may lose the game. There is also a risk you may make a mistake that really matters significantly to one or a number of your teammates. This occurs in all types of team play. So what?! It is just part of the learning curve. In team play, these decisions happen quickly, and the process of deciding to take risks on the playing field or court becomes second nature. Much like other life skills developed in team play, the more you play, the more comfortable you become. The more comfortable you become, the more confident and successful you are in the face of risk. The experience becomes familiar and is no longer viewed as threatening.

This is where play becomes so valuable. Few activities in life provide repeated opportunities to try, risk, learn and succeed – without long-term, significant effects on relationships, careers and self-esteem. Yet at the same time, these learned skills can make a huge impact that carries over into other areas of your life. The more you succeed in small ways, the more you will find the confidence to take on greater challenges – in play and in life.

Working together – for you

If practice makes perfect, then a team environment provides the ideal atmosphere as you learn to stretch your limits and excel. Several factors contribute to this:

Sports Teaches Educator the Rewards of Persistence

I started with track in seventh and eighth grade. It was not really competitive, just a couple of meets and you got your foot in the door. I went to a relatively small high school, where I was considered a track "star." During my four years, I amassed many honors and medals in sprints and long jump and went to state finals each year. Because of this record of success, I was invited to attend a track camp at the University of Michigan one summer.

As a child growing up in Michigan, I had always dreamed of attending the University of Michigan. Fortunately, I had the grades to attend, but knew that I wanted something more. I approached the track coach and asked if I could walk on to the track team. What could be more amazing than earning a varsity letter from the school of my dreams?

My freshman year, I worked hard on the track. I was not the best runner on the team, but I was the only long jumper. I ended up meeting my best friend that year; she was a freshman walk-on in high jump. We trained together, hung out socially and ended up placing in a few meets – but it wasn't enough to earn a letter.

I followed my summer training regime, coming back to a surprise in the fall. Due to budget cuts, walk-ons were no longer allowed to work out with the team. We had to make up our own practices, wrap and ice our own injuries, and get to meets on our own. My best friend and I decided we were going to show the athletic department that we would persevere, even without their assistance. Many other walk-on athletes simply quit, but we worked harder than ever.

Despite the obstacles we had to overcome, my friend and I both scored in more meets than we had our previous year. Our coach recognized our commitment and, in our junior year, he allowed us to be on the team and receive all the same benefits as the scholarship athletes. We had our best year ever, traveling across the United States with the team and earning enough points to get a varsity letter and letter jacket.

My senior year, I was still a walk-on athlete, but was able to stay with the team through all its practices and travels. A big highlight was placing in the top 10 in the long jump at the Ohio State University stadium during the Big Ten outdoor meet. That, along with other performances that year, gave me a second varsity letter.

I still have my plaque, my letter jacket and other mementos from my track years tucked away in the attic. But I also have something more that I carry with me every day: life lessons. I learned about the value of a team, knowing I had to fight harder than any of the others to continue to be a part of the group. It also taught me to be a part of the team, knowing when to speak up and when to stand back. I learned how not to let individual differences get in the way of the larger goal, and how to deal with people of different personalities. I learned about taking risks, competing to win, and how to be a leader when times are tough.

Most importantly, I learned about pushing myself beyond my limits. I could have stopped when I was at the front of the pack in high school, but I pushed to be a walk-on in college. I had to push harder to continue to compete when the support to walk-ons was cut. I pushed yet again to letter not once, but twice, for the school of my dreams. Every day, I apply this experience of persevering to win, in spite of obstacles.

Today, I'm a physical educator at a Maryland private school for students in pre kindergarten through eighth grade. My message to the kids? It does not matter who wins or loses; we are here to play and have fun. I know that if I can get them in the game, I can help them build the confidence to consistently push their limits and accomplish things they might have never known possible.

Stephani Kolevar
Physical Education Teacher

- Everyone on the team sees what you are doing at all times. You cannot hide your less-successful experiences – and neither can your teammates! This helps you keep it real and grow comfortable with being a work-in-progress.

- Each of your decisions and actions is experienced not just by you, but by everyone on the team. This means you are constantly exposing your level of commitment, willingness to take risks for the team, and determination when things get tough. In addition, it ensures that you will demonstrate your raw, true potential.

- Every day, you have the opportunity to work with a team of people who are looking to grow and succeed together. This boosts your motivation and creates synergy. The group's collective efforts to improve make each team member better than she would otherwise be as an individual.

With clearly defined goals, roles and expectations, a team can perform at high levels. For example, on my softball team, each woman clearly knew her role. There was never a question of who was responsible for first base, second base, and so on. This clear understanding was developed through countless hours of practice, as well as a commitment to the team. As a result, we exceeded the expectations for our positions individually, and extended ourselves to lend a hand to our teammates when needed. By being a member of a team, we can try new approaches and techniques, challenge ourselves to strengthen our skills, develop new strengths and take informed risks – which often leads to surprising rewards.

Push yourself, encourage others

As a member of a team, there are never-ending opportunities to stretch yourself – even beyond what you believe you are capable of accomplishing. Never stop challenging yourself to grow. Even athletes at the top of their game continue to reach beyond their limits. For elite athletes, this means breaking their own records by split seconds. Those split seconds can mean the winning margin.

Winning in sports may not be your goal. But giving yourself the chance to do the things you want should be a lifelong goal. Your goal may be to play for fun, for exercise, for companionship or for a new experience. Learning to enjoy team dynamics and the inevitable successes thereof, as well as overcoming difficulties and challenges, are worthy goals in and of themselves.

Most of us don't know what we are capable of accomplishing until we go beyond what feels comfortable or natural in our lives. You must get more comfortable with pushing outside your limits in play, in order to duplicate that ability to take worthwhile risks in other areas. When you learn to push beyond the boundaries from the past, you will no longer miss opportunities.

In the end, you have the choice on how far you extend yourself. You have the choice to play. You have a choice to contribute to the team. You can choose to push yourself to be your best, or you can choose to sit on the sidelines. Start small. Use team play as a means for trying new things and building your confidence. When others quit in the face of challenges, you persist. You have more in you than you can even imagine.

Playbook
As you challenge your personal limits, keep these tips in mind:

1. **Identify your goal.**
   Think about additional activities you would like to experience and enjoy.

2. **Assess your starting point.**
   Seek out an opportunity to join a team, then develop and learn at a pace that challenges you while building your confidence.

3. **Get out there and get in the game.**
   Set aside concerns or inhibitions you have about the contribution you may make to a team and focus on the potential you have as an individual.

4. **Constantly set a new finish line for yourself.**
   Once you reach your goal, reshape it. Remember, no one is in

your way but yourself. Don't settle for the status quo.

Workbook
Ask yourself these questions to encourage reaching beyond your limits:

1. When was the last time you pushed yourself outside of your comfort zone? What did you do and how did the situation turn out?

2. What were the lessons you learned from that experience?

3. Have you replicated that experience a second time?

4. Are you able to push yourself, or are you better off when others assist you in raising your own bar?

5. What process do you use to help yourself reach your potential?

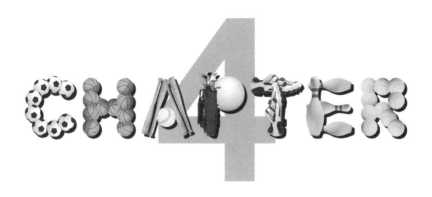

Taking Risks, Opening Doors

In the last chapter, we explored how pushing beyond personal limits can create significant opportunities. In this chapter, we will extend those limits a bit further by learning to take calculated risks.

What's the difference between stretching limits and taking risks? Here is an example to illustrate the point. Imagine that you have never played on a team. The very thought to play on a team may be well beyond your comfort zone. Now imagine you have made the decision to join. You are taking a risk stepping out assertively, reaching over and above your comfort level in a public way.

You might push yourself to join a team on the county or city league. Here you can learn the basics and have a good time. As your comfort grows in your new space, you may take greater risks when circumstances present themselves. You may want to steal a base or make a cross-court pass. These are calculated risks.

Risk-taking is marked by three distinct characteristics:

- A high level of the unknown

- Your own vulnerability

- A minimal level of control over outside variables

The unknown is always a risk. Should I join? Will I be successful? Should I take the chance? By taking a risk, I feel vulnerable and exposed. These are logical and normal responses that many contemplate when taking risk. Taking risks requires you to extend yourself just a bit further, outside your limits, to be successful.

As a member of the team, you may see an opening on the field or court. It's up to you to get the ball to the net or the goal! You take charge and make it happen, even if a successful outcome is less likely to happen.

There are varying levels of risk. Off the court, at work or at home, risks usually increase with higher levels of financial commitment, larger numbers of people involved, or increased personal exposure. Yet the things we perceive as the greatest risks often create our greatest rewards in life.

Changing your perspective

It is difficult to prepare to take risks if you have no experience in taking them. It is a huge question and unknown for so many. A risk may seem small or ordinary to most, but depending upon your degree of experience and confidence, the hesitation may be greater.

Typically, perceived risk and fear are products of the imagination. In other words, you might amplify the actual risks of a particular action. Let me offer an example from my own life experience.

As a businesswoman, I make many decisions both personal and business-related. I completed graduate school and became an entrepreneur, just 12 short years after obtaining my degree. I was confident in my decision-making, taking action and sticking to a plan. Then one day, a dear friend asked me to contribute a chapter to her book. The anthology, *Wise Women Speak*, is a collection of stories and life lessons. I knew I had something to share, at least she told me I did. I also knew that I had a support team available to help me in whatever capacity I requested.

But there were so many unknown elements! How would my experience translate into a compelling story that others could enjoy? Did I want the exposure and to reveal my vulnerability to others by sharing personal feelings, thoughts and experiences? How would I be received? An outsider might say; Where is the risk in writing about your business acumen and experiences? It certainly doesn't appear to be a risky project or proposition.

Although the risk appears slight, it is the images that are magnified by the risk-taker that must be reduced to overcome that genuine fear and threat. While my ultimate decision was to write the chapter, the decision to proceed was a tough one to make.

With great risk come great rewards

The risks that you sow are in direct proportion to the rewards you reap.

Why is that, you say? Imagine you have taken on a project with foreseeable obstacles. Despite the significant roadblocks, you manage doing the project well.

Upon completion of the assignment, you take pride and expand your self-confidence. These character-builders would not have developed as extensively if a lesser challenge had been mastered.

Consider my chapter in *Wise Women Speak*. I had been successful in business and was very comfortable sharing my story as a speaker. I knew I could engage an audience and inspire people through the stories I shared. Yet, I did not know how rewarding writing this chapter would be.

After the book was published, others thanked me for sharing my story. It was then that I had an epiphany. I could reach so many more people if I wrote, in addition to speaking engagements. The writing experience gave me the courage to take a new risk and write the book you are reading. I never dreamed of writing a book, but with this relatively small hurdle behind me, I had new motivation to go beyond my perceived limits.

On the flip side of reaping rewards is a relatively little-known fact: Avoiding risks may generate a negative impact by creating a party of missed opportunities. It may actually have a negative impact. Playing it safe is not always playing it smart. Sometimes risk-taking is necessary if you want to succeed.

Different women, different risks

Risk is defined differently for each of us.

Prior to launching my business, my career path had focused on education and service. I never imagined owning a business until I had the idea for Corporate Fitness Works. At the time, becoming an entrepreneur didn't appear to be a huge risk.

Today, with decades of business experience and acumen to look back on, I view my initial actions as incredibly risky – for my career, my pocketbook and my family. So why did it feel so natural at the time? Why wasn't I daunted by the task?

Again, I must credit my experience and background in sports. I learned to face risk straight on, manage it and succeed. I had evolved to develop a strong, natural self-confidence based on past experiences on the athletic field. As a result, I was not afraid. It was passion, the strong belief in myself and the mission that drove me.

Each of us is different, and it is important to assess where you are with your own comfort level of risk. Start small. Rate yourself on a scale of 1 to 10. A rating of 1 means that you simply get into the game. As a 10, you aspire to be a team leader, captain, coach or mentor exuding that intangible that everyone recognizes. What is the entry point that feels most comfortable to you? Begin there.

Next, identify the obstacles that keep you from taking risks and opening new doors. These barriers may be less than you imagine them to be. Remember, your mind is a powerful tool and you may often harbor fear that does not exist in reality.

Finally, learn to grow more comfortable by taking mindful risks. Take them in increments; no jumping in with both feet first. By taking these risks in small steps – but not indiscriminately – you can try new pursuits without the feeling of being overwhelmed to try new and different things. Risk-taking must be evaluated within several contexts.

Ask yourself these questions:

- What are your past, relevant experiences?

- What is best for your team?

- What is likely to work well?

- What is the cost of not taking the chance?

Take an honest look at the risk and make sure you are keeping perspective.

Are the barriers interfering with your willingness to take risks being overemphasized? If so, remember that taking small steps toward your goal may present instant rewards and gratification, constantly building your confidence as you near a successful end.

Once you decide to take the risk, don't look back; think success. Follow this formula:

1. Create a positive attitude. Look at every risk through the eyes of someone who sees the glass as half-full. Once you choose to play, don't focus on the risk, hone in on the opportunity and its rewards.

2. Exude a calm confidence in your actions, reactions and your interactions with your team. When you feel a bit tentative, use self-talk and reassure yourself and your team by embracing this attitude proactively.

3. Even though you may feel that engaging others exposes your vulnerability, do it anyway. Ask for help, advice and involvement from those you trust. Remember, it is through team play that we accomplish more than we think we can.

Learning to take risks in sports builds confidence to take us to the next level and reduces the fear of failure. In business and in personal life, the same applies. It is risky to speak up, voice your opinion or introduce a new idea, especially when you have no frame of reference, no experience and only fear. Women can start small and practice leadership skills by chairing a committee, leading a project team or running a fund-raising activity, and using the new-found confidence they acquire to take their game to the next level.

As in life and play, taking risks helps women achieve successful relationships and business goals by stretching their abilities and capabilities in a way that engages others and offers a reward beyond just their own personal achievement.

Playbook
As you consider taking new risks, keep these tips in mind:

1. **Risk = Opportunity.**
   What makes every risk worth taking is the opportunity that lies on the other side. Keep this in your sights. Those who can quickly acknowledge a challenge that is presented with this mindset will move on to reap greater rewards in a more timely fashion. Remember the old saying, "There are two ways to climb an oak tree. You can climb it or you can sit on an acorn and wait for it to grow." Need I say more?

2. **Start small.**
   Begin building your confidence by extending beyond your comfort zone in situations you perceive as less risky. You can minimize your risk by making decisions that impact mostly yourself and are seen only by a small group. Make decisions with little or no financial implications. Your success is bound to build your confidence and prepare you for the next opportunity with a larger role in the game.

3. **Know yourself.**
   Be aware of your risk tolerance. Every person has a different comfort level with risk that can be attributed to their experiences, as well as their genetic makeup. The goal is to stretch your boundaries but not too far outside your confidence zone. Working within your tolerated level of risk will allow you to function at your best. Your success in the small stretches will build your confidence to take on the larger ones.

4. **Engage others.**
   Identify teams that are supportive of your proposed risk. At lower levels of risk, these people may not be affected much by your success or rewards. They can, however, be there to support you emotionally and provide a sounding board to give advice. As the level of your chosen risks grows, the level of engagement by your team members will expand as well.

Coach Gives Back to Community What Sports Has Given to Her

I have played sports since I was 7 or 8 years old. Tennis eventually became my primary sport, but I was originally a swimmer. As a troubled youth, sports helped me focus my energy, gave me purpose and kept me grounded. It also expanded my world, because I was introduced to a great deal of cultural diversity growing up and playing sports in Los Angeles.

Playing sports encouraged the development of my educational skills and ultimately paid my way through college. I was injured my senior year in high school. These physical challenges that resulted from sports participation gave me strength, courage and determination. I was lucky enough to benefit from Title IX, which created so many opportunities for me to receive athletic scholarships. I also earned money through my college years by teaching tennis.

Education became my focus during my undergraduate years. I first thought that I would be a chiropractor. When I was awarded an assistantship in my graduate program as an assistant coach at the University of Miami, this was the beginning of my coaching career. Ultimately, I made education my profession and now teach at the university level.

To a great extent, learning to take risks and overcome obstacles in team play shaped my willingness and ability to take other risks that have ultimately turned into some of the most significant experiences in my life. As a coach, I was recruited to Alabama State University, where I coached both men and women. I was unique there, both as a female coach to a men's team and as a Caucasian in a predominantly African-American school. At Alabama State, not many female students had sports as their focus. As a result, I recruited players on campus and taught them to play and win. Most of them went on to successful professional careers as everything from biologists to attorneys. I still keep in touch with many of them.

While I feel that I have been able to have a unique impact in young people's lives, I still think that sports have given me much more than I could ever give back. Sports brought me to my current profession in which I continue to have the opportunity to impact young people and continue to learn and grow along with them.

Andrea Pent
Professor of Sports Management

They may invest time, money and talent in your cause and, at this level, they will reap the rewards of your success as well as the success of the team.

5. **Be prepared.**

The decision to take a risk should be an informed decision. Before you commit, confirm that you have the resources necessary to be successful. This includes your personal skills, the most current and accurate information surrounding the risk, support from others and financial resources. Wise planning may take a minute or it may take a month, but it will inevitably contribute to a successful experience.

6. **Check your mindset.**

Focus appropriately on the opportunities and rewards, while keeping the risk in perspective. Are you confident that you will be successful in reaching your goals? Are you ready to engage others in whatever level of support you need? Are you prepared to share the rewards with your team? If so, you are halfway there.

7. **Decide and act.**

Make decisions and act with confidence to move forward with your challenges. Once you have identified your interest or passion, assess the opportunity and engage others at the right level. Again, don't look back.

8. **Be flexible and realistic.**

Don't be afraid to modify your plan as you uncover new information. We can all appreciate when life deals us the opportunity to run straight up the middle and score. In reality, you will need to bob and weave with some fancy footwork to win. Not only might the process look different, but success also does not always look the same as you once envisioned. This could mark the beginning of new experiences.

Workbook
Ask yourself these questions to uncover the right risk to bring rewards:

1. What does your risk history look like? Describe the most significant risks you have taken in your life and ask yourself what the outcomes were.

2. Take inventory on what benefits taking risks in your life has given you. In retrospect, what would you do differently?

3. Is risk-taking easy for you? If not, how can you change your perspective and give yourself permission to begin taking small risks in the near future?

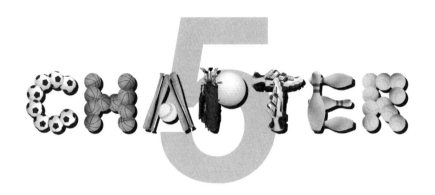

Find Your Team

We've investigated the reasons why women don't always jump on the team-play bandwagon. And together, we've explored stretching limits and taking calculated risks. Now it's time to take your first big step: Find your team.

Play looks different for each of us. To find the right team, where you feel comfortable enough to learn, grow and stretch, you first must define play for yourself.

I sometimes wonder how different our culture might be if we collectively emphasized the importance of play. What if we were taught, as children, to walk a mile each morning and night, just as we were taught to eat meals at the table? What if we expected, as adults, to play for an hour after work? What if we shifted the norm, adopting a mindset where play is as routine as brushing our teeth? Unfortunately, we do not live in this dream culture. As a result, the fundamentals of play are subject to an adult learning curve. Before we can play, many of us must overcome barriers, find support, and quash fears associated with self-confidence and failure, personal desires, priorities and needs.

I witnessed this exact issue in the community where I live. I bought a volleyball net, installed it in the common area of our neighborhood, and recruited a family that liked volleyball. But just because I built it, it didn't mean others in the neighborhood came. It reminds me of the movie, "Fields of Dreams"; remember the voice in the movie that constantly repeats, "Build it and they will come." It takes a lot of work to convince people to come. I began inviting more people to come play. This year, I will invite teams of six to participate from the neighborhood and play.

Volleyball is a great adult transition game. It can function as a catalyst to help adults overcome many of the hurdles, meaning it helps grown-ups overcome many of the barriers and resistance to play. First, it requires that players constantly play different roles and positions in the game, rotating from front row to center to server. Further, it requires true teamwork where multiple players can be required to hit the ball before it is permitted to cross back over the net. Finally, not every shot has to be a winner. All you have to do is get a hand on the ball and keep it in the air, so that a player in the right position can get it over the net. No one sits on the sidelines; we all rotate into the game.

Putting play first

Getting into the game, however, can be a struggle when juggling priorities. The last time many of us remember planning our schedule around play was in high school. In a school setting, your classmates and friends often encouraged you to schedule play into your routine. For some it was intramurals. We then finished school and embarked upon professional and personal roles, and our schedules got tighter and other barriers arose.

Where did the time go? Don't worry, you're not out of time. There is always time to play. You must appreciate that play is an essential component in your life regardless of age, gender, experience or lifestyle. You must change your mindset and attitude, learn to manage time and have the desire to play.

Yes, playing on a team takes time and emotional energy, but the rewards and benefits are immeasurable. In the end, the experience repays your investment exponentially. You feel better, accomplish more and find new passion. There is nothing like being on a team where everyone contributes and feels good about the part they play. When every player knows the goals, knows what is expected of them and is a part of the success of the team, it is an experience like no other.

Searching for new communities, new forums for play and new playmates make us all feel vulnerable. This can be exacerbated if you have past life experiences that make memories of childhood play difficult to overcome. For some, it is the memory of "picking teams" that prevents them from playing team sports. The experience of standing in a line and hoping you will not be the last one chosen – which is synonymous with being publicly called out as unwanted – it can bring back horrible memories. For others, the training and testing for fitness in school created negative feelings toward group physical activities. Someone has to be the last to cross the finish line when doing laps or counting sit-ups. As other children who finished earlier watched you struggle, you could only hope that you would never be put in that position of public humiliation again.

But those bad memories are long past. There is a time and place in life to build a new experience. That time is now.

We have all heard the saying, "You are never too old to learn." I believe you are never too old to learn or re-learn to play and have fun. I didn't play racquetball until after I completed graduate school; then I was hooked and still play competitively after some 35 years. No matter your age, playing on a team can be the best experience of your life. You don't have to be the star. You just need to play, enjoy and learn everything you can from the team interaction, the chance to compete and, most importantly, the chance to be your personal best while having fun doing it.

Get in the game

How hard is it to find a team? It's not hard at all. In fact, it is easy! Just look around and there they are.

There are walking groups, swim teams, bowling leagues, junior varsity and varsity teams, and recreation guides for just about any kind of sport you can imagine. You can check out your city or county recreational programs to find so many opportunities.

Sit down and spend some time thinking about yourself and your relationships. Consider these questions:

- How can you change your life by building relationships and managing change in an environment of play?

Attorney Redefines Winning and Becomes an Athlete in Her 50s

I always had a competitive interest and the desire to be a part of team sports, but the opportunity to participate kept avoiding even my best efforts.

Because I grew up prior to Title IX, there was little opportunity for girls to participate in sports, let alone excel and compete. Our only venue was physical education, where the logic of including all children in a way that helps them be a part of the play had not yet taken hold. The scene may be familiar to some of you. First, the most athletic girls were chosen as team captains. Then, in front of the entire gym class, all clad in one-piece, cotton snap-up gym suits, they selected their teams. You can imagine that selections were often based on qualities like popularity, size and athletic ability. Being small, I was usually one of the last selected. Not exactly the best invitation to get in the game and play! The remainder of the P.E. class went accordingly, with the select few throwing the ball to one another and playing as a team, while those of us who were left over just tried to stay out of the way.

It was the track unit in gym that gave me the opportunity to compete and helped me realize I could be good at a sport. I got my first taste of success when I accomplished the goal of one mile around the track on the first day. This became my competitive outlet, but it did not present the opportunity for a lifelong team sport. Running sustained me for many years until my joints started talking back. I needed a new venue in which to compete.

Living in Philadelphia, with its many waterways, turned me on to the idea of rowing. I gave it a shot. Much like my childhood experience, the results were not great. I had little training and quickly capsized the boat. It seemed that rowing was too daunting for me. However, life happens as life will, and I was diagnosed and treated for breast cancer. Who would have thought that this very trying experience would open new doors for me in terms of team play?

It was the distinction of being a breast-cancer survivor that provided me with my first sincere invitation to be part of a team. I was invited to a "learn-to-row weekend" for survivors, sponsored by WeCanRow DC on the Anacostia River in Washington, D.C., and it was then that I began my journey as an athlete. My success and wins may have seemed small to some at first, but with each milestone, I drew on my competitive drive, and each goal accomplished was my win.

First, I had to learn the language: port, starboard, ratio, catch, release, finish, and the components of the stroke. Next, I had to adjust my inner clock to waking at 4:30 a.m. Then, I had to toughen my mind to endure rowing when the cool or wet weather and the choppy water threw challenges at me. Could I do this? Was I strong enough?

Less than one year after the "learn-to-row weekend," I joined the Potomac Boat Club Women's Masters Team. My first team sport...at age 54! I love being part of the team, learning to row in unison, matching my body movements to the woman in front of me. I love the rhythm, the discipline, the sunrise. I love the hard workouts and seeing my erg scores and times improve and my fitness levels soar. I love the excitement of the regattas, especially beating a boat rowed by younger women. I sometimes wonder what it would have been like if I'd had the opportunity to compete on a team as a young girl. In the end, I am thankful that I was able to keep my competitive spirit alive and, in spite of setbacks, continue to seek a team sport. I'm thankful that the silver lining to my cancer was the opportunity to be part of a team of dedicated women athletes. This is my win.

Ellen F. Kandell, Esq.
President, Alternative Resolutions LLC

- What type of Parks and Recreation league would you consider joining?

- Is there a team at work that plays basketball, soccer, kickball, softball or volleyball, for which you could make time in your schedule?

- What is preventing you from engaging and improving your skills in a way that builds you and your team?

Look around and find others with whom you can form a team. In the beginning, you may come together because you wish to learn a new sport, hobby or activity – or re-introduce one you have not played in years. Once you get in the game, you will invariably find others who have similar interests to your own. You will find individuals with similar skill levels, schedules and interests.

Sometimes teammates are able to serve as skill coaches and teach, and other times you must learn on your own and motivate yourself to improve. Some teammates will move on quickly, while others will decide to spend more time playing together and possibly expand into other group activities. Playing well together is a product of the support your team members choose to give each other. It is also a gift that gives back to you in kind. A team identity is often defined by the support, dedication and encouragement that team relationships always develop over time.

The team experience helps you become your best as an individual, while also giving you:

- the "high" of team success

- pride in what you bring to the team

- a newfound focus on your individual strengths, as opposed to dwelling on weaknesses

The experience of succeeding as a team applies to family, marriages, relationships, work groups and community groups. "Playing" puts you in the position to consider and incorporate the ideas and opinions of others in a way that ultimately helps make you feel successful and fulfilled. To sum it up, working on a team is a thrilling event.

I met a woman who learned how to play tennis in her 40s when she joined an informal league. Now she takes vacations with her teammates and has formed strong friendships. But when she started, her intent was just to play tennis. Anything is possible once you get out there and play the game. Remember, you don't have to be good to get started, but you have to get started in order to be good.

It is never too late to get in the game. No matter where you are in life, there is a team for you, a game for you to play, and a team that will give you support and provide a venue to have fun.

Playbook
Here are a few things to keep in mind when considering which teams to join:

1. **Play with others.**
   Find your preferred interest in play or your suppressed desire with play. Playing and teams go hand-in-hand.

2. **Engage others.**
   Life is about relating to and being with people.

3. **Develop relationship skills.**
   Building relationships is the foundation for life.

4. **Change is inevitable.**
   Adaptation is the course for success.

5. **Seek others and form teams.**
   Our relationships grow through networking.

Workbook
Here are a few questions to ask yourself as you consider who you want on your team.

1. What comes to mind when you think about teams and teamwork?

2. What experience have you had working with, observing or playing on a team?

3. What skills did you learn or observe as a result of being on a team?

4. What might inspire you to join a team?

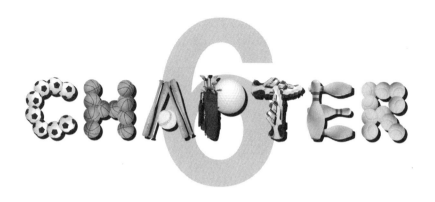

Practice Makes Teamwork

As you practice, so you play. It's an adage I heard over and over from my brother. It is so true and has made a huge difference in how I perform.

When I was a child, we played after school until it was dark outside. We squeezed the most we could out of every last second of daylight. This continued through junior high and high school, until the type of play changed. When I grew older, I spent my time in after-school practices or playing games with an organized team. My childhood play evolved, and I was better equipped to apply what I learned as I progressed to each new level.

This story is the same for many children. Childhood play evolves into formal practice as they grow, creating a natural and positive progression that challenges them and develops their skills. Organized team practices also help children develop non-athletic skills that serve them well throughout their lives.

Even if you have never taken part in team play, you can still identify with the value of practicing. Think back to something you practiced tirelessly until you got it right. Most people remember the repetition involved with learning to ride a bike. You may have started out slowly on a tricycle, later moving up to training wheels. Then, one day, it was time to take off the training wheels and take on a new challenge. Yes, you probably suffered a few bumps and bruises, but you persisted.

What was your motivation to try riding without training wheels? Did you see someone else riding a bike and want to play the same way? Children love to learn new things that they see others doing. This incentive helps them learn to walk, talk and read, as well as to learn a long list of other life skills. They try repeatedly and work to improve. In short, they practice.

The motivation in this and any other new challenge in life needs to be intrinsic. You are the one who ultimately needs to decide that the rewards are worth the risks. Yes, your parents may have been running alongside holding the back of your bike seat. But in the end, they had to let go. You were the one who decided to keep pedaling.

It was worth it. The practice paid off, and the feeling of success as you rode away down the street was life-changing. It represented success, independence, risk and reward. When you appreciate both practice and play, you begin to feel good not only for the fun of the game, but also for its rewards.

As an adult, you can duplicate the liberating and exciting experience of riding by yourself. There are so many other accomplishments in your life that come from practicing until you get something right. Haven't you heard that practice makes perfect?

Repetition builds confidence

Practicing isn't just for kids. As adults, we need to incorporate practice into every aspect of our life. Take an inventory of your own practice habits:

- When was the last time you practiced or planned for interactions in your personal or professional life?

- How do you know what your team members need from you, and what you need in return?

- Are you prepared when your team member needs backup?

The key to answering these questions lies in repetition as well as shared experiences that come by way of practice. Unfortunately, in many life situations, we don't get the opportunity to rehearse. People don't practice for success in the workplace. There is the expectation that they can just go out there and play to win.

In contrast, with team play you learn an entirely new concept: "as you practice, so you play." Each individual gains experience through repetition and practice, and for each person a unique set of resulting life skills is created. No two people come away with the same end result of practice and play. At the very least, you stand to build confidence while learning dedication, commitment and perseverance. You can even minimize the fear of risks and maximize your ability to overcome mistakes.

One of my most memorable practice experiences occurred while I was playing second base for the nationally ranked Plain American Softball Team. I felt privileged to be playing with this caliber of women and loved every minute of it. The team challenged me to be my best, while also valuing the contributions I made to the group. We practiced drills for every situation that could possibly occur in the infield. Our goal was to field all grounders and fly balls, without errors. Why? If we could practice with no errors, we could perform to that same high standard in a game.

During these drills, each player had to be prepared for multiple game situations. We never knew where the coach was going to hit the ball, or how she was going to hit it. We had to be on our toes and ready at all times. At first, practices were intimidating. I do remember how nervous I was; there was a lot of pressure to do well. But eventually, with repetition, I grew to the point that I wanted the ball to be hit to me. I felt prepared. It was such a great feeling. As my confidence increased, I grew to know exactly where to throw the ball in any situation. I was always ready to play.

Any kind of practice makes perfect

Historically, women have not benefitted from the concept of team practice. Team sports were prioritized for young men, but not necessarily for girls and young women. Of course, there were elite leagues for exceptional male athletes, but as a rule, practicing as a team is not a common experience for the majority of women today who did not play sports.

Instead, many women can relate to other kinds of practice: learning to play a musical instrument, singing in the choir or rehearsing for a play. As a child, you may have dreaded practicing the piano every day. Or you may have been motivated by what lay on the other side, when the notes flowed and playing music became uplifting, stimulating or relaxing.

Unfortunately, outside of sports, our society does not typically place a high value on team practice. As adults, we fail to grant ourselves the permission to practice in non-threatening environments. We forget to prioritize practice, build teams and play. I'll use myself as an example. I loved sports and practiced every day in high school. As I got older, other priorities took hold. Even my travel teams only practiced a couple of days a week. In recent years, I found a group that plays racquetball three to five times a week. This team was the motivation I needed. It encouraged me to get out and play more often, and I can't tell you how much I look forward to it. The interaction, practice and play pushed me to improve my game and motivated my desire to play. I have learned new strategies and refined my game as a result.

In fact, team practice always brings added value through skill development. For example, by working together toward a common goal, teammates experience positive social interaction, support and motivation.

The opportunity still exists for each of us to get in the game. Engaging in team play and practice could be something new. It could be something you have set aside in recent years. It does not matter what activity you play; it simply matters that you do something. This comes easier if you do not take this decision too seriously. Remember: It is just a game. There are many safe activities in which you can be involved. Try something new, practice and, as a result, achieve a new level of confidence and fun. The skills practiced and developed can be applied to other experiences in life. In your personal and professional life, this discipline and practice translates into time management, balanced budgets, well-planned meals, public speaking, supervision, leadership, facilitation of groups, attentive parenting and solid friendships.

Getting down to business with the team

What is the best approach to develop through practice? It all starts with finding the right team.

When a team arrives at the practice field, each player should know it is OK to push beyond their own limits and try new techniques – without an emphasis on the fear of failure. It takes great levels of mental energy to manage fear or avoid new challenges. It's much easier to put yourself out there, trying some new approaches, building confidence and doing something well.

When you practice in play, you learn to handle surprises successfully when it matters. You also build other skills and a mindset that serves you well in many dimensions of life. Practice is synonymous with commitment and dedication. Practice is the physical and mental preparation for "the game." Practice is the safe place to make mistakes and to learn from each mistake. Practice serves to impact the end result for the better. Whether or not the outcome is a win, tie or loss, preparedness and practice gives you a better feeling about your contribution to the game.

Frequent team practice develops and enhances relationship skills. Issues that affect your everyday relationships have probably surfaced on the playing field. Thus, practicing as a team, the stick-to-it-ness and the issues that teams must overcome, prepares you for situations at work and life experiences with family, friends and co-workers. All personalities that typically present themselves on a team are inherent in any group. There will be the leader, the motivator, the supporter, the cheerleader, the one who lacks commitment, the one who is always right and likes to be in control, the one who corrects the coach, the one who focuses on self over the team, the one who needs to be reassured, the one who needs to be humbled, the one who resists the rules, and the one who wants to complain and change the boundaries. There are going to be underachievers who want to quit early, and overachievers who work overtime.

In the end, while you develop the skills found in working with different personalities, you feel the most successful when others in the group complement and support your skills, values and style of play. You also need to do your part to develop as an individual and build the team's confidence in you.

Developing the best you

In the end, practice isn't just about developing experience. It's about developing the best-possible you.

A commitment to practice can be life-changing. Think about children and young adults with aspirations to be Olympic athletes. In some instances, these children practice so much they don't have time to play without purpose. This commitment to practice, however, makes the difference in the form of split-second wins and record-breaking performances. Do you remember the 1980 Winter Olympic Games, when the U.S. men's ice hockey team pulled together and won the gold medal? That was an amazing time not just for the team, but for the entire country. Even those of us who are not typically spectators of ice hockey were glued to the television, cheering the team on. This underdog team had the world mesmerized by its success, which was the result of hard work and countless hours of team practice.

A similar drama was played out by the U.S. women's soccer team. The gold medal came down to a free kick, and the entire nation was rooting for victory. It was the practice of that one kick, over and over and over, that would make or break this team and deliver the gold medal.

What makes the Olympics different from professional sports? Could it be the knowledge that these competitors are not perfect and are frequently not paid; they are simply committed to giving everything they have to preparation and practice, all building up to one single goal? U.S. swimmer Michael Phelps and other gold medalists instantly became role models for children and adults alike. This is not because of their victories alone, but also for their commitment to practice and perfection.

We may not be Olympic athletes, but we need to give ourselves permission to play and improve our performance for the sense of pride that comes from commitment. Prioritize practicing something new and committing to your own improvement. There may be no lights and cameras, but you will see yourself as successful, continually coming back for more.

In addition to learning from elite athletes, we can all learn a lesson from the thousands of children who play Little League sports each year for the first time. "T-ball" is more about practice and play than it is about winning. Parents cheer the batter for getting up there and giving a few hearty swings, even if the bat never connects. This is what keeps kids coming back for more.

But what if you missed the window of opportunity to play in leagues where participation, rather than winning, is celebrated? Start small. If you need to start practicing at home by yourself, so you can feel natural and comfortable in your play, begin there. When you are ready to extend yourself, find those who are interested and willing to take the same risks or have taken similar risks before, and those who value progress even if it is not attached to winning.

Find venues for adult first-timers. The city parks and recreation department is a perfect place to find the practice sessions and mentors you need. Look for others who you enjoy and recruit them into something they might not have otherwise considered. Women by nature are inclined to seek social support. Take advantage of this tendency when it comes to play. Your support may be a personal trainer, or it may be a neighbor. Just find someone and go play. Don't wait another year, another month or another week.

As I was preparing to write this chapter, I saw a coach at the airport with her team. She was wearing a T-shirt that, in just three words, said what she knew to be the essence of success: Desire, Determination, Dedication.

What do these three Ds mean to you? If you want to learn, you will practice. If you stick to it, you will improve. If you prioritize play and practice, your dedication will pay off.

My advice is that you apply this concept to your everyday life. Take small steps to improve in ways that help you do things you really want to do. Pull your dreams out of the box and decide how to make them happen. Plan a practice schedule for improvement and advancement, focusing each day on fulfilling the dream.

P-R-A-C-T-I-C-E

The word "practice" can be used to define the true value of experience:

- **Preparedness:** In a team sports practice, preparedness means drills that cover every possible situation that could occur in a game. By becoming adept at physical drills, you become more prepared to respond in other settings, such as the boardroom and the community center. Being prepared can apply to even the smallest details of eating, sleeping, and mental and physical preparation. Preparedness can impact you in each phase of your life.

- **Repetition:** In softball practice, I would field up to 100 ground balls during a practice. Over time, the "right" response became a natural response. Repeated practice helps you perfect subsets of skills, which add up to success. What skills are already a strength for you? Practice those, as well as additional skills or techniques that could be referred to as your weak spots. Repeat

Woman Builds Lifelong Relationship Skills and Friendships Through Team Sports

My life has been shaped to a great extent by the relationships I formed through team sports, particularly during many years of practice. I learned so many things by playing softball as a child and in college: how to get along with others, teamwork, perseverance, patience and cooperation.

Through weeks and months of practicing and working toward a common goal, my teammates and I formed long-lasting bonds much stronger than those with an officemate, co-worker or neighbor. Some of my 30-plus-year friendships and relationships come from playing sports as well. I still stay in touch with my coaches and athletic trainer, who are retired now. I also get together with former teammates, but not as often as I'd like.

I now have a doctoral degree and work in middle-school administration. I love my career and the opportunity to reach children and young adults. In my role in education, I have come to recognize that not everyone had the same life-shaping team play experiences as a child. If you only participated in P.E. as a required course, you may not have had the opportunity to experience team play at its best. The administrator at the school where I work had a terrible experience in all of her years of P.E. As a result, she avoids team sports to this day. She is, however, supportive of the girls' and women's sports in our school and understands that her childhood experience has limited her as an adult.

I, on the other hand, had an amazing experience with my P.E. teacher. We did not have an organized athletic program at my high school, but my physical education teacher took a great deal of time with us outside of class. I still remember this physical education teacher meeting my mother halfway between the school and our home (a distance of about 30 miles) to help with transportation, so that I was able to stay after school and participate in informal tournaments between classes. I cherish these memories.

My goal is to give back in the same way my mentors gave to me. I deeply believe in the power of teamwork. I try to impress upon young girls that they should be involved in team sports, so they will have the same opportunity as I did to build relationships through practice as a team. One of the programs I organize and deliver is a national girls' and women's sports day which is held each year in conjunction with National Association for Girls and Women in Sports Day. I begin by talking about the opportunities available to young women today. I try to help the students understand that this has not always been the case, even in the recent past. I explain the history that has opened so many doors for girls and women through Title IX, and through both athletics and academics, and I speak to them about commitment and link this to the sports experience. The girls then have an opportunity to participate in a variety of traditional and non-traditional activities.

I hope every girl and young woman has the opportunity to experience team play, whether competitively or non-competitively. Through practice and a team commitment, she can build relationships and personal skills that will last her a lifetime.

Dr. Jane Lynes
Middle-School Assistant Principal

your success in play until you can visualize yourself executing the skill perfectly:

- **Attitude:** Positive mental preparation is one of the many benefits of practice. Don't wait for the opportunity to present itself. Go out and create the opportunity to practice, improve and succeed. If you can't be on the field or court, you can still practice in your mind and spirit. Women have to give themselves permission to take the time to play and practice what is important to them. They need to visualize themselves winning and succeeding. As you think and as you practice, so you play. Believing in yourself is an extension of having the right positive attitude. Eighty percent of winning or being successful is your attitude.

- **Confidence:** Building confidence comes from succeeding in small increments. The more you practice, the greater the improvement; the greater the improvement, the greater the passion; the greater the passion, the sooner the success. Celebrate your success to convince yourself that your practice paid off. The experience and feeling of success can play out in many areas of your life.

- **Time:** Being your best means taking the necessary time for refinement. If you are committed to a project, activity or goal, you will spend time with it and derive the most benefit. What you put your money and time into is what you will prioritize. It does not have to be long hours at a time. Your practice can be in short bursts. The more time you commit, the better you become and the more you enjoy the process and the outcome. Soon, you will find that you don't have to schedule time. Rather, you will seize the time as it presents itself.

- **Initiative:** Your desire needs to be at the core of your decision. It has to come from within. For some, the desire may come from a motivation to win. For others, motivation may result from a desire for companionship. Whatever your desire, it is important to set your goals based on your unique definition of success.

- **Commitment:** Don't expect someone else to push you to perform. If a goal is important to you, you will be committed. There is no excuse for not being fully engaged at practice if you have made the commitment. You would never even consider missing the opportunity to play and, in turn, improve. You simply show up, give it your best, and feel good about the time and effort. Team members depend on you to be there. This expectation and your commitment are the keys to success.

- **Excellence:** It feels good to succeed. This does not mean being the best. It means being better than you were before. Define your own excellence and celebrate when you reach the desired outcome. Always strive to exceed your expectations and feel good about pushing yourself to go beyond what you ever thought was possible. Stretch your limits.

Playbook
Here are a few additional thoughts to keep in mind when considering the value of practicing with a team:

1. **Start today.**

   Take on a new team-play adventure. How do you know when the "right" moment presents itself? Start today. Only you can make it happen for yourself. You have so much to gain from this new experience. If you believe it is important to live for today and live out each moment to its fullest, then you will embrace this opportunity to play for so many reasons. Why wait for an invitation from someone? You create the opportunity for yourself and others to experience team play at the level that is just right for you.

2. **You are never too old to learn.**

   When you stop learning, you stop living. So what are you waiting for? Allow yourself a few minutes each day visualizing what it would look like to play something that you have always wanted to. What does it feel like? What emotions did you display? With whom did you share it? What feeling did it leave you with? After experiencing this mental exercise for a period of time, try it on for size and make it a reality. You may be surprised at the results.

Discover the joy of practicing. Keep practicing so you will reap the joy of feeling good about yourself and working through new situations. Whether you practice to improve your skill, better yourself as a person, build up your own confidence or minimize your fear of mistakes, or just practice for fun, it is all positive. The benefits of practice and play are there; embrace them.

3. **It takes a community.**
Surround yourself with others with whom you have fun and enjoy spending time. It is amazing what you end up doing with people you love being with. Think about the community you can build for yourself. Who will you invite to be part of this experience? It takes time to build your personal mixture of people. The end result is deriving the greatest benefit from the shared experience. Again, you deserve all of this. It just takes time and making the process a priority in your life. So what are you waiting for? Start today and make a list of those close friends and family members with whom you wish to play.

Workbook
Ask yourself these questions to determine if you are really taking advantage of the opportunity inherent in practicing your skills.

1. How do you practice skills in your life now?

2. If you have practiced on a team, what skills did you learn that you are using in your life today?

3. How can you incorporate a practice schedule into your current job or situation?

4. What skill would you like to develop that you might not have thought possible for yourself?

5. Have you thought about keeping a journal to reflect upon your experience?

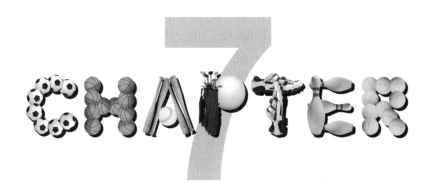

Think On Your Feet

While many stand weighing the opportunities presented in life until conditions are just right before acting, others go out on a limb by betting on themselves and experiencing the rewards of success.

If practice makes perfect, it also creates major advantages for those willing to invest both the time and the effort. Why? Because those who practice learn to think on their feet. That means reacting to a situation and making a decision quickly and confidently. You need to know when to pass the ball, to steal a base, to rely on your teammates, or to battle on your own and score. This insight and learned behavior can be very important on the sports field, in the business world, or in the many roles you play in life. Women have had particular challenges in the area of decision-making, particularly fast decision-making. To reach your potential, you must grow more secure handling whatever comes your way. This includes projecting self-confidence about your decisions. As a girl, you were expected to defer to your parents' decisions. As a student, you were to follow your teachers' directions. In past generations, it was common practice for women to defer to their spouses. This is less true of our culture today. As a family member, community member or employee, you must be prepared to think on your feet, make a call and commit.

I observe the differences in the behavior of my employees. Those with a history of playing team sports are better prepared to make decisions with confidence. When critical thinking comes into play, they are more comfortable explaining and defending their points of view and recommendations. Ultimately, those who present their position with confidence are rewarded with the support of their peers and company leaders. Further, they exude the same confidence as they follow through and deliver. They are accountable for their decisions and actions.

But the benefits don't stop there. Team members unknowingly apply the same type of critical thinking skills quickly and effectively – on the spot – when engaging in other life experiences. When playing team sports, you are constantly making decisions and immediately act on them, both during practices and in games. Once you have made your decision and called the play, there is no time for waffling. You make a commitment and put your whole heart and soul into the play you have chosen. If you pause to second-guess, you risk making the wrong decision and consequences occur. It is too late to go back. This is a lesson we learn by playing sports: make a firm decision and follow through on it with confidence.

Sometimes, the split-second decision will be correct. Sometimes, it will not. As you become more polished at making quick decisions, there will be more and more success stories to build your confidence. Consider, however, that there is something to be gained even if the play does not turn out as anticipated. For example:

- Through lessons learned, you come to understand that you can only predict so much. Invariably, there will be surprises. When conditions change, you learn to shift mid-play to adjust to these surprises and even pull out a win. These decisions must be immediate. These skills can be applied to life experiences when unexpected variables come into play.

- You learn not to take it personally – a huge step for women to overcome. Often women have difficulty separating a project or task from personal feelings. With experience from thinking on your feet, you come to realize that this is all part of playing the game. You are not perfect, and you are not going to make the right decision every time. You also learn that a less-than-ideal decision is not the end of the world. Instead, you develop the ability to quickly process the experience and move ahead, leaving further reflection for a later time. This is a huge lesson for all of us to learn in life. Try not to take things personally, because you cannot control the actions of others. Whether on the court or the playing field of life, it's all about playing the game the best you can and letting go of the rest.

Thinking as a team

Making quick decisions on the field or the court is a risky business. To encourage team members as they develop their fast-thinking skills, team members and coaches need to be supportive. This sets the tone that encourages players to act decisively.

Team members must embrace the idea that you can make a quick decision and lose a point, yet still win the game. At the same time, team leaders need to encourage risk-taking and decisive action, and give constructive feedback that empowers players to think independently.

In earlier chapters, we discussed the importance of choosing the right team. Act decisively when choosing your team. Settle only for a team that shares your values and embraces your unique skill sets, as well as your potential for growth. Making a commitment to a team empowers you to be your best, while making the most of your time, energy and positive commitment.

Consider the following questions when making your choices to join a team:

1. Will the team support you?

2. Will the team present an environment for your personal growth?

3. Is this a team you will commit time to? Do you have a desire to do your best as a member of this team?

4. Will you embrace the values of being true to your word and your team? Will you deliver even if there are unexpected variables along the way?

Once you choose the right team and are ready to move forward with confidence, you should always be prepared to think on your feet. With doubt or without, you have to make a move. Although doubt may exist from time to time, you must be prepared to think quickly and make that move. Don't be afraid of doubt or failure; those who achieve a lot are those who seek it while conditions are not the most favorable. Those who wait for the most favorable conditions, rarely win. Don't worry, the outcomes are going to be okay. At the game's conclusion, you will quickly take personal inventory of your performance as well as receive feedback from your teammates, coaches and mentors.

If you have experience in team sports, you can appreciate first-hand the benefits of fast thinking. But, if you haven't yet had this opportunity, let's consider some other areas of life where you may have developed the skill of thinking on your feet. For example, parents commonly make quick, decisive moves in addressing their children. We have all observed a parent whose child asks permission to visit a friend or buy a new toy, and the parent hesitates. When they pause and fail to give a decisive answer, the parent's hesitation opens the door for the child to believe a "Yes, I can" is achievable. Teamwork is thinking and acting decisively. In contrast, the parent who responds quickly and with confidence is more likely to receive deference from her child, without negotiation.

In other situations, at work or at play, your opinion may not be requested. What if the role you typically play is to follow the decisions of others? What if you are not usually given authority to think and act on your feet as a general rule? In that case, team play can present opportunities for you to break that cycle and to build your confidence and self-esteem. Find a team that is supportive, one that gives you space to develop and expand your decision-making capabilities. Let the team selection be your first priority. Don't spend years in roles that fail to provide you a platform to apply your good critical-thinking skills. Rather, think and act decisively.

In a preferred team environment, members work hard to provide the right balance of responsibility, authority and accountability within the team. Great leaders seek opportunities for team players to feel challenged. However, if the team is large or if the leadership is preoccupied or bogged down with other issues, you may not be called out and asked to grab hold. Don't wait for someone to hand you the ball. Be proactive, take charge of the situation, and make it happen. You will never know what is possible unless you take action and try it out. I always say, "What is the worst thing that could happen?" Don't be offended if they are not interested or they simply say no. But if you never ask, you will never know.

Support goes both ways

Sometimes, thinking on your feet means making a decision and taking the lead for the team. At other times, it means stepping back and supporting the decisions of others. When others on the team are in a decision-making position, be prepared to support them in the same way you hope to be supported if the roles are reversed.

In other situations, the ball will fall between two people. True team players think on their feet to "call it," or say that they are in the position to field the ball. They must also be prepared to assess the situation, listen to their teammates, step aside so that the other player has plenty of room to manage the situation, and then move into a backup or support position.

Can you imagine how this same scenario would play out in the workplace? Both trust and confidence must flow both ways, and sometimes the best play will be to defer to a team member's ability to make the call. There is no harm in seeking help or letting someone else take the lead for the benefit of the team. Those who are true team players inherently understand this concept. It becomes second nature for a great team member to relinquish responsibility when someone else is stronger in a certain skill or area of expertise.

Growing comfortable with a fast pace

With practice, thinking on your feet becomes natural and comfortable. Regardless of who has the primary responsibility, team players develop skills and innate reflexes become automatic. Through self-discipline and practice, athletes learn to trust their instincts and perform in challenging situations. In practice, the best coaches force the repetitive practice of this collaborative work.

As children, we want to be everywhere and anywhere that the ball is on the playing field. If you have ever watched a soccer game played by 5-year-olds, you can see the group swarming around the ball and moving in harmony down the field. The ball is like a magnet, and the little players

Team Sports Teaches Business Owner How to Think on Her Feet and Use Decisive Action to Win in Life

I have played sports all my life, beginning with playing in the street and trying to keep up with the boys. In middle school, I was on the girls' softball and gymnastics teams. Then, I went to a small, newly opened high school that had only two grades, which enabled me to participate in more sports than most: men's track, women's swimming, tennis and cheerleading teams.

I came from a family where sports were not considered important in a girl's life. I say this without judgment, and I am sure my dad understands it comes from my passion and desire to encourage other young women to get their dads to their games. While I was growing up, I did not have my dad at my sporting events because he thought he needed to be at my brother's events instead. I felt like I needed to work hard and play with tremendous drive to get recognition. This need to excel meant that there was no time to play it safe. I had to think outside the box, trust my instincts, and surprise the opponent and our spectators with my quick judgment and resulting success.

As an adult, I am an avid golfer and play with men. I also worked for a period of my career in NASCAR. The large variety of the sports I played, as well as my desire to keep up in men's sports, taught me how to think on my feet. Especially because I spread myself thin across many sports, rather than perfecting one sport or one position, I needed to call on my judgment without hesitation to react in practice and game situations.

This experience set me up to work in a man's world by learning to be a business partner and team player with the opposite sex. Men play different games than women do, and it was helpful to be on their team. They move fast, play aggressively and don't over-think their decisions. They are also less likely to look back. Win or lose, they support their teammates' decisions and move forward to learn from their mistakes.

While I had many opportunities in sports, I also had some unique challenges that reinforced my tendency to forge ahead and compete without hesitation. When in gymnastics at a young age, I fell off the balance beam. It was assumed that I had a broken leg, until I was diagnosed with bone cancer. I continued to work out as my treatment would allow and ultimately won this battle as well. If I had paused to consider what having cancer potentially meant, I might have stopped short. In the end, this attitude to follow my instincts taught me that anything I put my mind to could pull me out for the win.

I am very passionate about mentoring young women who can benefit from my experience. I still get e-mails from young women I have not seen in years. They will reach out and thank me for encouraging them in ways that led to their fulfillment and success as adults. I have an entire wall of more than 4,000 business cards I have collected over the years that remind me daily of the lives I have touched.

In the end, it is not just the legacy of a passionate competitor that I hope to leave. I want people to remember that I kept paying it forward…without hesitation.

Cindy Sisson Hensley
President, HOPSports

don't appreciate the concept of staying within their assigned zones.

Through development, maturity and experience, a player learns to stay within assigned boundaries and be ready when the play comes to them. This growth development assists each of us outside of play as we make conscious decisions to either get in the game or step out of the way. Also, in team sports, you learn appropriate levels of engagement that complement the goals of the team.

For a team to work together with speed and efficiency, players must learn to communicate and act decisively in concert with one another. The ability to make decisions as a team is just as important as making decisions quickly and effectively as an individual. Obviously, this too can be developed in the team-play experience. When you play, as an individual and in concert with others, you need to make the decisions that are best for the situation and the team. Consistent communication plays out in non-sports settings, such as executive boards or council meetings where everyone must be on the same page if progress is the desired result.

Transferring your new skills to other forums

Through practice and play, the repetitive process of taking decisive action becomes easier. After working on this skill in play, you will be in the position to confidently act and make decisions with ease in other aspects of your life. Just follow these simple rules of engagement:

- Do the advance work: Being prepared means being the expert on the information or topic in a variety of situations that may present themselves on short notice. You will need to make informed decisions to be fully effective on a team. Sometimes, the best decision will be to take the lead. Other times, you should back another team member as he or she develops a plan of action and execution.

- Plan for the expected: Have a plan in place for the most-predictable scenarios. Within your scope, have a clear understanding of what your appropriate move should be. Know that sometimes the situation will be unique and take you by surprise. You will lean on your own experience to make a plan on the spot, given what you know.

- Engage others in advance: Communicate your plan to others who may be impacted by or involved in your decisions. This can be done in your role as the team leader if you are in the position to determine the plan. It may also be accomplished in your role as a team member who can bring proposed solutions to the discussion for brainstorming and collaborative decision-making.

- Practice the desired response: Know your role and replay it in your mind until it becomes second nature. Stand in front of the mirror and communicate your plan with clarity and passion until you feel you have convinced your team.

- Keep an open mind: What are other possible scenarios that you may not have imagined? Use your experience to quickly coordinate strategies for success. Being open-minded will help you better understand that you will not always have all the right answers.

- Act decisively: When the time is right, make a commitment to your action plan. Stick to it and execute it to the best of your ability. Don't second-guess yourself. Be flexible, but not tentative. Be prepared to make mistakes, persevere and move on, inspired and the wiser from the experience.

Playbook
Here are a few things to keep in mind as you enhance your ability to think on your feet:

1. **Let go of old paradigms.**
   Tentativeness based on past experience or others' expectations can make it difficult to make decisions. It is not always up to someone else. When you do take the lead, be mentally prepared to think and act decisively in that team leadership position. Remember, your opinion as a team member matters – so express it.

2. **Be accountable.**
   Whether the decision you make leads to the perfect outcome or some portion thereof, be confident that you made the best decision you could given what you knew at the time. Be accountable to your team members. There are always things to be learned and new scenarios to add to the long list of possible outcomes. If the decision was yours, own it!

3. **Trust yourself.**
   Make a decision, go with it, and see what happens. Many people avoid making decisions because they do not want the outcome to be bad. How do you know how good you are unless you make a decision? Take a chance on what you think is right. You will never know your capabilities unless you go with your gut feelings when the opportunity presents itself. Others will learn about your ability once you step out with confidence.

4. **Know your role.**
   If you want a safe place to ask questions and make on-the-spot decisions, a team-focused culture must be in place. Your role on a team must be clearly defined, so you know when it is appropriate for you to lead in the decision-making process. If your defined role is to lead, surround yourself with team members who want you to succeed as part of the team's success. Don't settle for anything less. This approach will ensure a friendly environment to ask questions while in pursuit of making informed decisions. Once

you have found the right team, let it be known that you are ready and willing to think on your feet and act decisively on their behalf – and that you are ready to be accountable.

5. Seize the opportunity.

On any team, some are comfortable thinking on their feet. Others, meanwhile, have great ideas but aren't ready to step up to the plate. Resist the temptation to hesitate. It feels good to take the lead; act decisively and enjoy success. Practice seizing small opportunities as a first step. Find new situations where you can apply these simple rules and build your confidence by making decisions and sticking to them.

Workbook
Here are a few questions for you to consider as you work toward greater comfort in thinking on your feet.

1. Think about a time you stood up and made a point in a department meeting, committee meeting or family discussion. What happened? How did you feel?

2. Do you have the confidence, courage or strength to speak your mind? If you do, what lessons can you share with another woman who wishes to reach this place in her life?

3. If speaking out is something you need to work on, what would help you become comfortable speaking up and sharing your knowledge and talents with others?

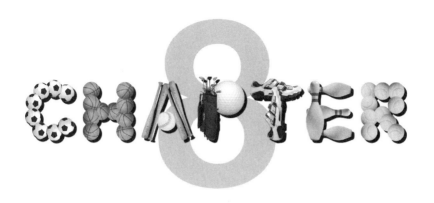

Learn From Your Mistakes

Every mistake is an opportunity, calling for someone to grab hold.

Imagine a young girl in school being told by teachers, coaches and parents that it really is OK to make mistakes. Even more shocking, what if these role models and mentors actually encouraged you to make mistakes in the hopes of accomplishing something extraordinary?

Suddenly, your world would be turned on its head. Learning something new would no longer be considered a risk. It would present nothing but opportunity. Sounds too good to be true, right?

Wrong. You can make that decision for yourself today. Decide that trying new experiences, even if they include making mistakes, is an important part of getting into the game of life. Making mistakes isn't just OK; it's critical to a successful life.

If you are pushing beyond your comfort zone, you are going to make mistakes. When you learned to read and write, you didn't know all of the words. Each time you tried a new book or wrote a new sentence, you read or spelled a few more words right. Remember when the teacher asked you to read aloud in class? This was probably one of your first experiences in taking risks. Sure, your mistakes were obvious to your peers. But chances are that the teacher quickly corrected any missed words, and you moved on.

Doing something new is all about gradually getting better and better at it. This is true when we take on our first job, our first relationships and our first leadership role. There is, however, a significant difference in how we tend to deal with mistakes made during our adult lives compared with the missteps of our childhoods. As adults, we sometimes spend more time and energy worrying about potential failures than we do brushing ourselves off and trying again. Our biggest mistake is that we constantly fear we are going to make one.

Don't misunderstand me. I am not implying we should define our lives by our mistakes. Rather, I am suggesting that we define ourselves by the lessons we learn. Being open to and prepared for mistakes means having a plan in place to process what has happened, learn from the experience, and minimize the possibility that the same mistake will happen again.

From mistake to opportunity

Wimbledon Cup winners usually get the ball back over the net and in the court just one more time than their opponent. Did they have some missed shots? Sure, but they stayed in the game.

Hanging in there is sometimes a success in and of itself. When you get in the game and choose to play, things won't always go well or turn out the way you want them to. It is your responsibility to take those lessons and learn from them.

I don't focus on mistakes. Rather, I remember past situations in order to avoid the same pitfalls in the future and to accelerate improvement. I acknowledge the mistake, move on and improve. Remember that the goal is to win the war, even though you might lose the battle.

Fans and team members celebrate overall success in spite of errors made during a game. The headline in a local paper doesn't ever read, "Loube misses four free throws in Friday's varsity game." Instead, the story tells who won the game, as well as what happened that was surprising and unexpected. Learn from this.

There is a list of clichés that tell us this message is not new. Pick yourself up and brush yourself off. Get back on that horse. Don't cry over spilled milk. While the message is not new, it is sometimes easier said than done!

Don't get me wrong. I am not suggesting you ignore the error or the missed play. But view those mistakes through the correct lens. If you miss free throws, everyone is aware of your mistake. The key is to take full responsibility and do something about it.

In the short term, you have to handle it alone. No one can help you recover from the mistake while you figure out how to finish the game. You are the one who will need to bounce back and prevent the mistake from happening again. You are the one to present yourself in such a way that others know you have things under control. Mistakes are nothing to get stuck on. You have a choice to pull it together and finish the event with success. Further, you can make your final free throw to win the game. You can do it; you simply have to put your mind to it and believe in yourself.

This is the real challenge, and if you allow yourself the opportunity, the lesson will carry you as you move forward. You can grow in confidence and become better as a result. To me, the key to turning a mistake into opportunity is to first and foremost own up to the reality that it was a mistake. Make the mistake – but learn from it. Then, take full ownership. Denial or coverup works in the opposite direction. It teaches us to brush things under the rug, and eventually the dust piles up. View your mistakes as useful stepping stones to a higher level of competency.

Learning from your mistakes requires that you share the experience with your team. This might be your colleagues, friends or family. It may be the people who were impacted by the outcome. Or, it could be those who are your support group or mentors, even if the mistake did not affect them. This is how we all grow. We learn from each other and our collective experiences and mistakes. Learning from the mistakes of others helps us gain focus in our personal decision-making.

In play, you learn to keep going, to take the next shot, to get back on the bike, and to try again. In doing so, you use the knowledge gained from mistakes made to improve and find success. There is no time on the playing field to beat yourself up, or sit and worry about things that didn't work out perfectly. After the swinging strike, the next pitch is coming down the pike. After the missed shot, the rebound is coming off the backboard. After the point, the next serve is coming over the net.

If you take advantage of your mistakes as opportunities to learn, you can use the knowledge gained from growth and greater achievement and reach for the impossible. In order to learn from your mistakes:

-    Recognize that there was a problem.

- Examine the root of the problem.

- Acknowledge what really happened and how it could have been handled differently.

- Identify the challenge and determine what your role was.

- Keep it together in the short term by keeping your head in the game. Don't let the mistake define you.

- Take full responsibility for your actions.

- Think of drills to practice in overcoming your mistakes. Your mistakes will then be of value to you.

- Honor yourself and what you are doing to learn from your mistakes.

- Exercise mental toughness along with physical preparedness.

- Identify opportunities to develop your own individual skills, as well as team skills.

- Remember that small improvements add up to big ones.

- Initiate new opportunities, in spite of the chance for new mistakes.

- Re-define mistakes as experience.

- Motivate yourself to achieve and raise the bar each time.

- Believe in yourself.

- Live out the new experience and apply it in other areas of your life.

- Celebrate your successes.

Winners take time to process mistakes and make adjustments, so they can improve their experience next time. Winning teams help and support each other as they turn mistakes into opportunities. Success-minded people do not get bogged down with their mistakes; they realize that mistakes are a necessary part of the territory and ultimately a part of tomorrow's successes.

Grow together as a team

Just as team play enhances the potential to push boundaries and take risks, working within the group also increases the chances for mistakes. Learn from them. Remember, you can embrace the opportunity inherent in taking risks, and the potential rewards, to a greater extent when you are working as a team. In team sports, if taking a risk means you don't quite make the play or win the game, the team still acquires wisdom and becomes smarter through its mistakes.

The team huddle and practice sessions are ideal venues for discussions and interaction. A team huddle would be great in many aspects of life, wouldn't it? Here we can each consider our role and how we can better perform, and then share the success or the challenge as a team. Through this approach, we learn to take responsibility for our own challenges as well as those of the team. We learn from our individual and collective mistakes and create a camaraderie of support, all the while building team relationships and unity. This is much preferred over tearing down the team, placing blame or dwelling on past errors. Just think about how many places in life we could apply this mindset!

When working as a team, we not only learn more and grow from our mistakes, but also from the mistakes of all team members. What a gift! Learning from others is equivalent to living the life of many, rather than the life of just one person.

Lead through mistakes

The best coaches view mistakes as opportunities for their team to learn and grow, both together and as individuals. Pat Summit, coach of the women's basketball team at the University of Tennessee, provided an excellent example of the opportunity to leverage mistakes. After being eliminated from the 2009 NCAA tournament, she had her team back on the court the next day. She did not have them sit out until the next season. Pat used this time to teach and to review for all to learn and grow while the game experience was fresh on their minds. It truly was a teaching moment for the entire team.

You need to find people in your life who look to find opportunities for you to get involved. It can be the neighbor who invites you to play on the recreational softball team or the co-worker who takes on a team project. Whatever the case, they need to be ready to support you just as you support them, including the mistakes you make.

For those of us who are mentors or leaders, it is critical that we develop cultures in which people can relax and extend themselves. In other words, our team members should not be afraid of making mistakes and instead should enjoy the process of setting and reaching for challenging goals. This creates an incredible feeling of freedom for the team. None of us is perfect. Always remember that mistakes are as much a part of winning as perfection.

In my previous role as president of Corporate Fitness Works, the co-founder and I used our experience in team play to create a culture where team members were invited to grow and supported in their learning. As a result, they exuded confidence and believed what the team could accomplish together. Part of creating this atmosphere was a series of meetings where team members' opinions were encouraged, considered and valued. One of the key messages in these gatherings was that it is OK to make a mistake. If a team member did make a mistake, he or she was expected to share with their supervisor, identify the lessons learned, and determine how to avoid it happening again. Finally, the team member had to be open to sharing what was learned with co-workers.

Lifelong learning requires that you push yourself to try something new. And that means the probability of getting only part of it right the first time. But, as you improve, you can hone your skills, gradually succeeding in more and more of the task at hand.

How limited your life would be if you let the fear and embarrassment of making mistakes keep you down. If you can learn to give more attention to your successes and victories than you do to the pitfalls and challenges along the way, you are bound to strive for more of the same positive experiences with less fear of making mistakes.

The most effective lessons in life are charged with the emotions of risk and reward. Pause in your reading and think about this for a minute. Think of a time that you felt like a winner. Reflect on the road that brought you to that victory. Did you stretch beyond your comfort? Did you have some challenges along the way that you worked through? In the end, did the success matter more than the rough road it took to get there? Chances are, the answer to these questions is yes.

Playbook

Keep these things in mind as you work to leverage and learn from your mistakes:

1. **We all make mistakes.**
   Don't try to be a perfectionist. Accept the fact that you will make mistakes.

2. **Mistakes are opportunities to learn.**
   You will make smarter mistakes in the future.

3. **Share your mistakes.**
   Go to the people who need to know and discuss what happened.

4. **Assess the lessons learned.**
   Take notes on the entire experience and make sure you make the most of it.

5. **Engage others who you respect that can influence your learning curve.**
   Create your own team huddle.

6. **Make a plan.**
   Find ways you can stay clear of making the same mistakes.

Workbook
Reflect for a moment and ask yourself these questions.

1. Think about the last time you made a mistake. What happened, and how did you handle it?

2. What would you do next time if the same situation presented itself?

3. What lessons have you learned from making mistakes?

4. With whom can you share these lessons?

5. How do you let go of your mistake and move on?

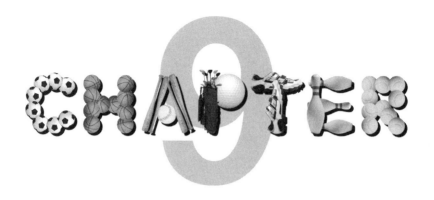

Compete to Win

Step on the court only if you plan to win.

A competitive spirit on the playing field doesn't always come naturally for women.

In fact, for most of us, competing is a process that must be learned. My goal in this chapter is to give you the permission and inspiration to make competition and winning a part of your life. Competing is synonymous with performing, and giving a top-notch performance is synonymous with winning. When you compete, you let your actions speak for you.

This translates in the workplace, as well as on the court. Women don't compete well in most job situations. Why is that? Well, perhaps the mentors and leaders of women have failed to validate the concept that competition is key to winning or being successful. Reflect on the chapters you have read so far in this book. Would you agree that most of the advice leads you down the path of building self-confidence, believing in yourself, and trusting that you have the skills and abilities to ultimately win or be successful?

To compete, you must be comfortable with the sensations of competing and the atmosphere of a competitive environment. You must learn that competing to win – whether individually or in a team sport – really is OK. To do this, you will need to gain some experience, build strength of character, and feel the excitement and exhilaration that competition provides. Once you get a taste of your success, an enlightenment occurs when you continue to apply a new-found competitive drive. First, however, you must eliminate any negative feelings associated with competing to win.

Digging deep

Competitive individuals must dig deep to find the right combination of traits they need to win. These may include:

- attitude

- emotional and physical makeup

- strength of character

For women, these are not always considered positive attributes. This creates conflict, as social norms encourage female behavior that is often contrary to the development of a truly competitive spirit. For example, has a male basketball player been told he should smile more on the basketball court? It happened to a young woman playing in the NCAA basketball tournament. Her concentration and intensity were interpreted as a display of poor sportsmanship and bad behavior. Do you ever hear a male being told in competition that their action or behavior was not "gentlemanly"? I think not. You do hear, however, that a female's action was not "ladylike."

Many women simply are not competitive by nature. That's unfortunate, as sports is a primary arena where women have the opportunity to learn to compete – yet relatively few adult women play sports. In addition, there are still women out there who feel the need to let the other "guy" win because it's the "nice" thing to do. I was fortunate to have a role model for the skill of competing graciously. My brother competed only by his actions, and never by his words. "You show your true identity as an athlete by your actions and commitment to excellence on the field or court and not by the words you speak," he would say. He knew how to harness this competitive advantage well and was exceptional in his performance.

Regardless of gender, age or any other inherent characteristic, development of a competitive spirit and drive is as important to peak performance as physical strength and skill. Strong will, passion and an unyielding persistence often provide a psychological advantage that reduces an opponent's advantage. I never understood why someone who wins the coin toss at the beginning of the game would give the opponent the first play or first serve. By doing this, you give the power and a psychological advantage. This occurs a lot in racquetball, when my opponent wins the coin toss and elects to receive. I am so excited to get control at the beginning of the game. The ball is in my hand and I have the first opportunity to score. If I had received, I would have had to get the ball back after running the risk that my opponent would score first.

Beyond a psychological advantage, competing to win is about projecting your intent to others. A family member recently approached me to talk about her application to graduate school. She was concerned that there were few spaces available at the two schools she was most desirous in attending. There were many candidates competing for those openings. Her mindset was to select a safe school, where she was assured of earning a place, rather than choosing to apply to the two schools that would create uncertainty and anxiety relative to her successful admission.

I asked her to slip into a new mindset, borrowing from her experiences as a competitive swimmer. "Picture yourself on the swimming blocks and imagine it's right before the race," I said. "At that point, did you worry about losing? Or did you prepare for the race with the intention of competing with passion and winning?" Of course, she answered that she never considered losing the race. She said, "I swim to win." Immediately, she understood the parallel between swimming and graduate school. Her job was to exceed the expectations of others by doing her personal best, and creating a tone – set with the expectation of winning.

Another conversation was with a college graduate now applying for a job. I reminded her that a few short years ago, she was the most valuable player on her high school varsity team and was the clean-up hitter (number four hitter in the batting order). I used that setting to illustrate the comparison to her job search. I explained that as an outstanding athlete, she excelled playing softball. I told her that when she got up to bat, she saw herself getting on base, not making an out. She immediately saw the analogy and it built up her confidence to take that same attitude to her interviews.

Once you find the competitive spirit, attitude brings it to life. After all, it's your attitude that demonstrates your intentions and sets you up to be a winner. It is a posture; it is how you carry yourself.

Winning truly isn't everything

What if you compete with all your might, but you still don't win? Does that mean you will never earn the title of winner, and that you are destined for failure?

Absolutely not! Many small wins along the path contribute to the greater win. These smaller victories can include:

- improvements

- recognition of a job well done

- application of learning from past experience

- a new-found confidence in yourself and others

- perseverance and mental toughness when things don't go as expected

You must be wise enough to choose the challenges that push you beyond your limits, while not setting yourself up for failure. You also must be real about what a win looks like for you in a given situation, and recognize each stepping stone as a success.

Let me use my experience playing racquetball as an example. I did not learn to play until I was in graduate school. I started slowly, and when I practiced to the degree where I was ready to compete, I found opponents who played at the same level. I moved up the ladder and took on increasingly challenging matches. Now, as I move onto new phases in my life, I realize that I am not in graduate school anymore. I set my sights on opponents who challenge me to be my best while remaining competitive in my age bracket and at my skill level.

Winning looks different to each of us. That means competing within your own limitations in a subtle, non-threatening and non-intimidating way. For some, competing to win means earning an Olympic gold medal. For others, it means just getting in the game.

Team play takes winning to new heights

Regardless of gender, competing as a team means striving together to achieve a common goal: to win! Competitive women are often labeled "aggressive." Some women also fall into the trap of taking this criticism personally. This perceived persona can be an obstacle in securing the respect of other players and serve as an impediment to personal success. In team play, however, women should feel empowered to embrace this competitive spirit as a positive trait. This focused, self-assuring way of thinking helps women pursue fulfilling experiences. It drives them to respect and believe in themselves, without taking criticism personally. It prompts them to seek others who have similar desires, ambitions and drive, who can support and encourage them to achieve their goals.

The true value of competition in team play and in life is seen in individuals reaching their goals. In sports, everything is geared toward competition. From practice to game time, the goal is to be as competitive as you can. You prepare to do your best, minimize your mistakes through practice and put attention to every detail. It is a conscious effort to do everything in your power to compete against your opponent. Whatever it takes is what you do. When it is time to perform, you are ready and prepared to win. It is the competitive spirit that brings that little bit extra to the game and ultimately delivers when others may fall short. It's that extra energy, drive, perseverance, commitment, confidence, determination and raw talent. It is going above and beyond what your competition is doing. In a final analysis, it's what separates the two teams. It is identifying what you want to achieve, focusing on it and then taking action consistent with our desire for success.

Reflect on a time and place you learned to put your best up against others and experienced the thrill of winning. It could have been on the field, on the court, in the science fair or in Girl Scouts. Where in your life did you learn to compete – or did you learn at all?

Competing and winning as a team makes for another kind of experience all together. When you are on a team, the common goal is to win. That's the bottom line. We don't just make the sacrifice to commit many hours of practice, sweat and tears for the little things. Yes, we want to play well. Yes, we want to have fun. Yes, we want to win and verbalizing it is OK for the simple reason that you don't want to let your teammates down.

Lyn St. James Finds Courage to Race in Team Sports

Beginning in seventh grade, I attended an all-girls school where we played different sports as part of our curriculum. The experience was somewhat of a shock. I was not athletic and was an only child who did not have role models of siblings in sports. This was long before Title IX. Thank goodness that I went to a girls school, or I would not have had an opportunity to learn to play. Even though I had no natural ability, I also had no choice. My best friend was an athlete, and she coached me through the experience. I went on to graduate with a major in business and later earned a certificate to teach piano from the St. Louis Institute of Music.

As an adult, I took up tennis. I was competitive, but I never really excelled. I used it as a social connection and took lessons before I would even consider playing with a club or joining a team. I enjoyed watching some sports on television, but really enjoyed going to car races. My husband and I both enjoyed the sport, and we found a club where we could both race. Just like tennis, I had to work hard to learn how to race. You see, I am competitive in spirit, but not necessarily physically strong. I was able to redirect this passion and competitive spirit in my own unique way.

Most people think of racing as an individual sport marked by great risk-taking. For me, it was neither of these things. Taking risks does not come naturally for me. I am scared to death of downhill skiing and even riding a ski lift. But when I am in control of the car, I feel like the risk is minimized.

One of the many lessons I learned in racing came after witnessing the death of another driver. I had to come to grips with the risk and decided that it was worth it. Teamwork is an integral part of a driver's success. Even though the driver is in the car alone, the driver needs a team to win. I see my team as a community that includes sponsors, the car, the mechanics and the pit crew. I see the driver as somewhat like the quarterback. It requires communications, leadership, and the expected team dynamics; it is up to you to deliver for the team, as well as yourself.

I started racing in 1973 as a hobby and eventually was able to enter my first Indianapolis 500 race in 1992, where I was the first woman to earn Rookie of the Year honors. I raced in seven Indy 500s over nine years and set a world record for women during the 1995 qualification weekend by reaching 225.772 miles per hour.

In 2000, at age 53, I was the oldest driver in the field at the Indy 500. My career in the sport led me to experience things I would have never dreamed of, including invitations to the White House to meet with Presidents Reagan, Bush and Clinton; and guest appearances on "The David Letterman Show,"

"The Today Show," CNN and ESPN. I was recognized by Sports Illustrated as one of the Top 100 Women Athletes of the Century.

At the risk of stereotyping, it seems that most women are reluctant to say they are competitive athletes. In addition, women are not good at sharing their personal success with others.

Yet if we do not share our history and our successes, we cannot help others find their own path to fulfillment. All paths to success are marked with the same life skills that can be learned in team play: dedication, risk-taking, extending beyond your perceived boundaries, learning from your mistakes and staying in the game against the odds. If I had not played sports, I would never have had the courage to start racing.

I have dedicated the later part of my career to helping other women. In 2001, I was given the Guiding Woman in Sports Award from the National Association for Girls & Women in Sports. I also served as the president of the Women's Sports Foundation from 1990 to 1993. In 1994, I established the Women in the Winner's Circle Foundation, a not-for-profit organization that provides leadership, vision, resources and financial support to help create an environment of opportunity for women's growth in the automotive and competitive motorsports fields. I have shared my story in three books, so that others can see how very far we can come by simply getting in the game.

If I could share one thought with girls and young women, it would be to stand up and discover who you are. Find your passion, and don't let anyone try to stop you. We live in a different era, where women can help women reach out and reach up. You do not need to be competitive by nature; you just have to believe in yourself and have a desire to succeed. This knowledge will be there even on days when you are not getting positive results. It is a core function. In racing, the term 10 tenths means 100 percent. I say, go 11 tenths – beyond your comfort zone – so you can get in the game of your choice.

Each of us has an arena from which we can reach out and influence the choice of young women to find a forum for team play and to apply all that they learn to experience life to its fullest potential. I have been given the gift of learning this in a sport not typical for women or expected for someone with my background. I want to give back, and I hope others will find a way to do the same.

Lyn St. James
Professional Racecar Driver

I have to share with you one of the most memorable victories in my life. It took place in Boston, where I traveled to play in a racquetball tournament with my sister. We played doubles and, due to the difference in our skill levels, my sister had to play at a higher division than normal for her. She held her own and I was so proud of her. We won that tournament and she played well beyond what she ever thought she could. She pushed herself and accepted the challenge to compete. She played as if we had been playing doubles together forever, not just for this one tournament. The win was bigger than the tournament because she had extended herself and expanded her potential to higher limits.

As a team, you complement and cover each other; you take personal responsibility, yet you celebrate success as a team; and you learn from mistakes without placing blame. If it is a real team effort, you win or lose as a team. You can take informed risks because you have practiced and played and built a resulting trust. The trust, collaboration and ultimate success you experience builds confidence. And all of this for what purpose? To succeed and hopefully strive to reach your ultimate potential!

Playbook
Here are a few things to keep in mind when learning to be competitive:

1. **Give yourself permission to compete.**
   Pay attention to what comes to mind when you think about competing. Be mindful of your feelings, both positive and negative. Take a moment to shift any negative perceptions so you can begin to look at competition as a good thing.

2. **Do the mental preparation.**
   Imagine how you would feel. Envision the outcome. Repeat the behavior so it sticks and begins to feel like a part of who you are.

3. **Learn to win as a team.**
   Recall the role you have played in the past on a winning team. Think about the gifts that you brought to the team that helped them win. Remember the experience and the feeling of victory.

4. **Translate a winning attitude into individual victories.**
   Think about how your own winning profile can translate into other parts of your life.

5. **Recognize the small victories.**
   There are small victories that we experience every day, yet we often fail to recognize them. Write down the next stepping stones toward your larger goal. When you accomplish one of these steps of success, recognize it, celebrate it and tally the win.

6. **Learn to enjoy the feeling of the win.**
   Visualize how you feel, illustrating the picture in your memory. Draw on it as you prepare to compete in individual or team sports. What could be so bad if it feels so good? Don't take winning for granted. Some people win so frequently that they fail to appreciate the great feeling of accomplishment. The positive energy from winning should never be overlooked. Always celebrate it and feed off of it for the future.

7. **Understand that the experience will be greater than you can imagine.**
   Trust in the positive results and allow yourself permission to keep the feeling alive. Would you feel differently if you won?

Workbook
Reflect for a moment and ask yourself these questions:

1. Have you ever had an experience where you competed?

2. If so, how did it make you feel? Did you enjoy it? Did the outcome impact your ability to want to compete again?

3. Does competing feel natural to you? Why or why not?

4. Do you feel there is a place for competition in your life? How would that competitive spirit impact your life?

5. What would inspire you to compete in the way you want to compete?

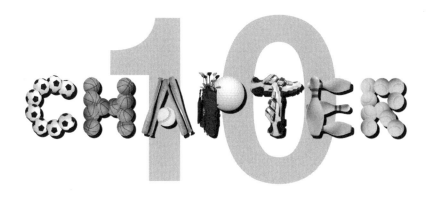

Celebrate Your Victories

Celebrating success is like celebrating life itself.

Winning feels great! With victory comes a combination of pride, satisfaction and pleasure. This is true whether you have won something beyond your control, such as a raffle, or something you worked hard to achieve. You might have enjoyed the satisfying feelings that accompany winning when you watched someone else experience the triumph of victory.

Think about times in the past when you have felt these sensations and consider these questions: Did you take the time to pause and acknowledge the victory? Did you share these positive feelings with others? Did you really celebrate, inside and out?

Celebrating is a learned behavior. To become more comfortable with the concept, it helps to watch other women as they delight in their victories. Unfortunately, there is no television sports channel dedicated to women, making it more difficult to find obvious displays of celebration on a daily basis. If we could witness the celebration, what would it look like?

Women would learn to:

- celebrate with the grace that is expected of us

- recognize others

- learn to accept compliments

- not worry about hurting or upsetting others

What are the parameters for celebrating with class? In team play, there are some simple rules to live by:

- recognize your mistakes

- celebrate the contributions of each team member, regardless of degree of participation

- celebrate your wins – not others' losses – and be humble

- elevate the success of others

Celebrating the success of others

In reality, most women don't rejoice in their own success. We may, however, applaud a victory for someone else.

Sometimes, of course, recognition of our own success is short-lived, thanks to the fast pace of our lives. More often, however, women do not stop and bask in the moment because doing so makes them feel uncomfortable. As a rule, women have been rewarded for modesty, as well as supporting others in their success. We typically have not been encouraged to push beyond our limits, expect to win, and then show pride in the victory.

I have been guilty of falling into this trap when uncomfortable receiving praise and also showing little excitement over a win. In the early stages of playing racquetball, a close friend came to watch me play a match. She watched as I paused to celebrate competitive points, ticking off point after point. But when the game was over, and I walked off the court victorious, my attitude was cool and casual. My friend asked me, "Didn't you just win that match?"

I responded, "Of course. Couldn't you tell?" I was surprised by my friend's reply. She said, "No. You do this all the time. You don't have a problem celebrating when you win a point or have a great play. But when the game is over and you've won, you downplay it. It's as if you don't want to draw attention to the fact that you've won."

Even I, with a lifelong devotion to playing and winning in sports, was not comfortable celebrating a win publicly. Like most women, I have a natural tendency to get excited about things – especially the small wins in a game. But when the big victory happens, women tend to deflate like a balloon, letting all the air run out quickly, and slip out of sight.

Celebrating a win with gusto, however, is the right thing to do. As a woman, I encourage you to take a new, revolutionary view of celebrating your success. If you take the time to extol your own accomplishments, publicly and without hesitation, it's not just for you. You provide a positive role model for your friends and family members, who also must learn to celebrate their own successes. You are providing a gift, to yourself and others, by celebrating a sense of a job well-done. The positive ripples from this celebration will flow into the lives of others, who will learn it is OK to party with success.

Team play is an excellent forum for learning to celebrate success – both individually and as a team. There are ample opportunities to celebrate for your teammates. They perform well at individual moments and as they bring home the win. Celebrating as a team is exhilarating. There are so many others who can share in the excitement. Rather than being a celebration of one, it's a party for your teammates as well. The coach and spectators exude pride in your success, too. Together you can high-five, hug, yell and jump for joy – on the field, in the stands, in the locker room, at after-game parties and even in your home with family and friends.

If women are unskilled at celebrating their victories in sports, they are even more inept at lauding their own accomplishments in other aspects of life. For most women, a victory is approached with a subtle and overly modest response. We are quick to acknowledge the success of others and downplay our role in the win. As a result, we miss out on the accolades – the happy, healthy and invigorating feelings that are the rewards that accompany the success of winning.

Celebrating team victories at work and at home is an essential and exciting part of life that creates strong personal bonds, builds a sense of camaraderie, and forms cohesive work teams and family units. What does this excitement look like to you? I want to encourage you to go beyond

Racquetball Player Inspires Others' Success by Celebrating Victories

For a racquetball player and personal trainer, celebrating means sharing experiences with family and close friends.

I was a tomboy growing up, skinny and gangly, but I could always run fast, so I always enjoyed competition. I gravitated to both music and sports, because I was exposed to both in my house growing up. I loved the joy of music in solitude and with an ensemble, and also the competitive aspect of sports. I ran track and played tennis in high school and a little in college. When I was introduced to racquetball, I found I picked it up pretty quickly as a transition from tennis. Racquetball became my truly favorite competitive sport from then on.

I started playing racquetball in my 20s and, at my now-husband's urging, entered my first novice tournament and won. From there it seemed I quickly moved through the divisions by winning tournaments at each level, and before I knew it, had become an Open level player.

I've never really talked to anyone about celebrating tournament wins. It's just something I do mostly with my family, who could not be any more supportive. It works both ways, because we all are super-supportive of each others' wins, and of course are there for each other during the frustrating outcomes as well.

I get a great deal of instant gratification, joy and satisfaction out of winning and the thrill of victory. One win in particular was especially exciting because it was an upset that came at a national event. I celebrated for only a split second on the spot, however. I have learned that my greatest satisfaction comes from sharing my victories with my family.

When I come home from winning a tournament, my husband will often have dinner and sometimes flowers waiting for me, and my boys, when they were younger, made congratulations cards. My family celebrates with me through phone calls and text messages throughout a tournament, and that has always kept me motivated to finish a tournament strong.

One particularly touching gesture came from a friend of mine who gathered up a few other women to create a beautiful framed memento of the tournament for me. It included the final score sheet, the draw sheet and a few reminders of the tournament. It blew me away that my friends took the time and effort to do that for me, and it hangs in a special sports room in my house.

There are others besides my sons and husband who celebrate on my behalf. My father was a tremendous supporter of women's sports in general, and of my racquetball. He was always the first one I called after a tournament. When I was named the Women's Racquetball Player of the Year for Florida, I dedicated the award to him because he had passed away just a few months before. He was an amazing man and sports fan who cultivated in me a spirit of competitiveness, joy and respect. My mom and dad have always been a big part of the celebration of a win for me: just making that phone call and sharing the tournament re-cap with them.

Some women are more comfortable than others talking about one person's victories. For those who open the door, I'm happy to share the experience. I certainly try to reciprocate when other women win, or move up a division, or beat a formidable opponent.

I try to help encourage women players to be really proud of their achievements. Most women tend to shy away from celebrating a win, and if we encourage each other and share in each other's successes, more women may try to aim for even higher goals.

Janet Tyler
Certified Personal Trainer

your comfort level. Get physical, tell others, throw a party — it is up to you how you do it. Just celebrate! On the job, send impromptu e-mails, or make calls or group announcements acknowledging when team members execute a winning proposal, host an exciting event or garner a customer's praise. In your family, plan gatherings, send e-mails, make calls or write online postings that create a tradition of sharing everyday good news. When you do this in a consistent, respectful manner, you can create a culture of celebration that is anticipated and admired by all. This habit creates positive energy and builds desire for, and expectations of, success.

Within our company, Corporate Fitness Works, we started a tradition called "A Positive." At the end of a meeting or workshop, we ask each team member to share a positive experience in both their personal and professional life. This ritual can contribute to a positive culture in any company. Don't wait for the awards ceremony at the end of the season to recognize the unique contribution each player makes to a team. When the awards celebration arrives, not one player should be surprised by what is said at the podium. They should already be fully wrapped in the recognition of their success and accomplishments.

Recognizing your unique wins

Once, I had the good fortune to coach a team that simply didn't have the necessary components to win. Why do I define these circumstance to be good fortune? The experience challenged me to recognize and reinforce my belief that winning isn't only a reflection of what is on the scoreboard. Because winning the next game was probably out of reach, I instead helped the team appreciate the more incremental wins it was capable of accomplishing. We established short-term goals to measure our success, and we celebrated the small wins. A win is a win, no matter how small.

Have you ever seen a team celebrate after finishing on the short end of the score? If a team was barely edged out in the final playoff game, wouldn't it be a revelation to see the players congratulate one another and smile, rather than shrug their shoulders and head for the locker room? Occasionally, the coach of a losing team will comment that her team did an amazing job by getting to the final round and playing a competitive game. These words are taken to heart by team members and others who, as a rule, appreciate the small victories as well as the ultimate wins. Unfortunately, this attitude is rare in our society.

Don't let that stop you from celebrating your own personal victories, even if they are not recognized by others. Success is not only defined by the win. It is defined by doing your best and improving on past performance. Sometimes, a "win" is as simple as performing some small task on the road to a larger goal. For some, success could lay in taking on a challenge that seemed overwhelming in the past.

Learning to celebrate your wins publicly is only part of the "feel good" about the competition equation. You must also develop the knack of how to lose with grace, being brave in defeat, extending yourself all-the-while to overcome shortcomings and achieve success. Victory looks different to each one of us. For you, a great win may be losing by one run to the team in first place or just making the decision to engage in team play for the first time after many years of playing the spectator role.

Sometimes, a win may not be familiar to you. Don't let that stop you from celebrating! When you are a winner, you should party like a winner. Each victory, no matter how large or small, has its own story, its own lessons to be learned, its own relationships. Appreciate it, value it, treasure it, embrace it. You don't know when this feeling will surface again. Further, celebrating has a ripple effect. It makes others around you happy and excited for you. You are not just celebrating your countless hours of preparation and dedication, you are celebrating for spectators, family and friends who have been engaged in your pursuit of victory. There may be many small wins along the path to the final buzzer.

Playbook
Here are some things to keep in mind when planning to celebrate success:

1. **Picture the win before you even get started.**
   Mental preparation is probably a greater contributor to success than physical preparation. Even the most talented fall short of victory if they do not have the right attitude and mindset to win.

2. **Recognize and celebrate the small wins.**
   Don't underestimate the reward and motivation that comes from celebrating small victories on your way to the bigger win.

3. **Define victory based on your personal goals.**
   Refrain from worrying about what others think. Remember that every small victory builds your confidence and brings you closer to the larger victory.

4. **Practice rules of common courtesy in your approach to celebrating.**
   A simple set of rules will go a long way toward making you feel comfortable with celebrating publicly and reinforcing this life skill.

5. **Recognize all victories.**
   Treat each and every little win like it is the first and the last. Take notice of the little or unexpected victories. Celebration takes practice and will become a habit when you get it right.

6. **Encourage others to celebrate their victories.**
   Take the initiative to plan and participate in victory celebrations. Share the enjoyment of celebration – it's contagious.

Workbook

Be a role model and share your own successes. When others share in your successful experiences, they are better able to envision their own possibilities. Ask yourself these questions as a way to become motivated and actively celebrate your success:

1. Think about the last time you celebrated a victory. What did you do? How and with whom did you celebrate? How did you feel during the entire time?

2. Do you plan how you will celebrate accomplishments before, during or after the task or project?

3. In the future, how could you help yourself and others share the excitement of and celebrate a victory or success?

4. How can you establish the expectation of celebration in every area of your life?

AFTERWORD
Play It Forward

Appreciate what you have experienced and learned. Give back. Help others to experience the same feelings.

By now, I hope you have come to appreciate how truly remarkable the impact of playing team sports can be in your life. This may be the result of trying something new and getting in the game for the first time, or you may have played team sports for many years. But did you ever stop to reflect and appreciate all that these experiences gave back to you? Whatever your situation, this book has attempted to reinforce the idea that it can be life-changing to get in the game, take risks, push beyond your limits, practice and perfect your performance, and celebrate the results in a consistent way.

Now, are you ready to take the next big step?

What if each of us could motivate and encourage at least two other girls or women in a way that gave them the same life-changing experiences? What if you could teach someone else that she, too, can play? Just imagine the ripple effects.

I recently met a mother who lived and learned the life-changing power of team play by supporting her children in team sports. It doesn't matter how you get involved. Rather, it matters that you embrace the value of team play, get engaged and play it forward. It is the active experience, not the level of play, that develops who you are today.

The power of mentoring others

What if a person in your sphere of influence could shift your mindset away from anxiety and into the belief that you are a winner? A person who would not push or cajole, but, instead, encourage and challenge you to compete to win. Just imagine the potential.

There is a fine line between those who act as mentors and leaders, and those who push others for their own sense of achievement. A successful competitive spirit comes from within but is nurtured by others who point out the opportunities and push us to motivate ourselves.

Mentors and role models are important for every participant or athlete, from the casual competitor to the professional. In my own life, as I focused more on professional goals, I drifted away from team play and into more individual athletic pursuits. As a racquetball player, I had to learn to translate the mindset of being competitive and winning from team sports to individual sports. It was my father who inspired me to make this mental shift. "When you step out on the court, you should expect to win," he said. "Otherwise, why are you playing in the first place?" Now as I step on the court I imagine playing my best and always paint a mental picture of success and winning. My dad's simple statement changed my life. Between my father and brother, I was fortunate to have such role models to help me understand the principles or guideposts along the way.

Mentors should always challenge you to do your best. But the most significant contribution a mentor can accomplish is to support and encourage those they mentor to celebrate their success. Players who appreciate how to win and celebrate their victories are consistently recognized and elevated to be team members in any discipline by their peers. A winner who exhibits skill, motivates others to play hard and celebrates the journey is always chosen the team captain by the coach.

As a team captain, you have the opportunity and are expected to help build your team's confidence and emphasize the principles of "one team." As a leader, you are in a position to drive the reaction of other girls and women in a way that fuels their desire to experience more of the same. If, in fact, you do secure a leadership role or have the opportunity to coach some day, you will be able to share your skills and the emotions of winning gracefully, and also share how to fully enjoy the moments linked to victory. You can leverage the experience of those you mentor to build their confidence, reinforce their achievements no matter how small, and instill in them a sense of value for pushing to do their best.

Have you ever been instrumental in helping someone perform to the best of their ability? It is a rewarding, stimulating and exciting experience. Just as you can get in the game and play, you can lead others in a positive way to do the same. Getting started as a mentor is easy. First, ask yourself these questions: Who are three people you admire as great leaders? What qualities make them great leaders?

While individual lists of these qualities may vary, most of us would agree that a mentor can inspire others with a clear vision of how things can be improved. An outstanding leader can also excite others to rally around their vision and make it a reality. They can motivate and encourage others by sharing their values and visions. In addition, they act as a role model by serving others and guiding individuals to surpass their own expectations.

Chances are, you have already played the role of leader and mentor in the lives of others. Pause and think about opportunities you have had to mentor, give back or help others. When I considered this question, I was able to make a list that was much longer than I expected. For example, I am fortunate to be an older sister. Growing up playing team sports, I was selected or elected captain for many of the teams I played for. I was a camp counselor, a coach, an instructor, a teacher and an umpire – not to mention an employer, a business owner, a committee member, an advisor and more. The list is endless. There are so many opportunities to lead.

Serving as a mentor in a variety of roles, I have garnered the reward of paying forward all that playing team sports has given me. By becoming a mentor, you can do the same. We owe it to girls and young women to give them the message that team play will impact their lives more than they can possibly realize. If you embrace the opportunity created for you in team play, you will be overcome with a desire to help others have the same experience. Whether you were lucky enough to have played on teams all of your life or you realized the potential of its impact later in life, you have the capacity and promise to point others in the same direction.

Bringing your experience and talent to the table is always an attraction to others who want to get in the game. We see this in professional athletes and Olympians who inspire children to swim, ski, do gymnastics, skate, etc.

To others, however, a role model who simply understands what it feels like to be a beginner is even more inviting. The opportunity exists for you to help others reach beyond their comfort zones and exceed expectations. To stand side-by-side with someone, assisting them to grow in play as a team or individual, is an investment of time. The rewards, however are electrifying.

Another opportunity to grow

Throughout the book, I have talked about team play as a way to develop your life skills. Leadership roles in team play provide you with a new level of opportunity to develop skills that apply in all areas of life. These include listening, communicating, delegating, solving problems and building teams. Leadership also gives you the chance to influence others and help them succeed. As a leader, you can elevate yourself by valuing your team members, rewarding hard work, putting your team in control of the outcome, and celebrating their success. Coaching creates yet another level of leadership by motivating you to accept new challenges and take initiative.

At this point, you may not think you have the skills it takes to be a mentor. I would like you to reconsider. Please review my list of the top 10 skills necessary to mentor effectively. Read this list slowly and carefully. Conduct a personal assessment to assure yourself that you already have what it takes to mentor. Do you:

1. …seek and value new ideas and feedback?

2. …trust and respect team members and opponents alike?

3. …recognize individual contributions and honor others' differences?

4. …ensure that all team members play a part in the win?

5. …maintain a positive and upbeat perspective?

6. …show a passion for what you are committed to?

7. …value and care for your team?

8. …walk in all team members' shoes?

9. …constantly keep the lines of communication open?

10. …remember to have fun?

In addition to these 10 qualities of successful mentoring, I encourage you to consider how closely you identify with some of the philosophies that are most important when taking on a mentoring role:

- Success is peace-of-mind, which comes from knowing you gave your best effort to become the best you can be.

- Help yourself and others strive to be the best they are capable of, remembering that perfection is a great target to shoot for, but oh-so-hard to hit.

- Be present, listen and show you care.

- Practice, practice, practice!

- It's amazing what is accomplished when no one cares about who gets the credit.

- Don't be afraid to say, "I don't know."

- Don't be afraid to ask questions.

- Help people feel significant, and they will make a difference.

- Believe in others as much as you believe in yourself.

- A mentor's ultimate goal is to create more mentors!

With these principles in mind, take another moment to create your own vision. Ask yourself:

- How can I get in the game?

- How can I encourage others to get in the game as well?

Consider where you see opportunities to influence and reach others. Is it the community center, the Jewish Community Center, the YWCA, your workplace or a school? Where do you have spheres of influence? Which groups would embrace your offer to help as a result of shared values?

Community is also important to the concept of "playing it forward." The definition of community has changed in our lifetime. Community size used to limit our relationships and interaction with others in team play. It used to be defined by our neighborhoods. Today, however, our teams no longer consist of only those who can ride their bike or walk to the same street for an afternoon of baseball. Competitive children's sports are played internationally. No longer are our co-workers those who sit in our office. Many people work "side-by-side" with others who live halfway across the globe. As community boundaries have given way to the power and ease of travel and technology, our ability to network with others has opened doors wider than ever before.

Leverage this power to find others in your own family, and then in your local community, who have common interests in playing team sports at the level that is right for you. Use a social networking site or blog post to find others with the same interests.

As you close this book, take any momentum you have gained on to the next level. Check out the online community at www.youcanplay.org, where you can find a network addressing the subject of play, its capabilities and rewards. Remember, play starts with the physical activity that will keep this generation and the next healthy. It builds contributors, team members and leaders. It strengthens us as women and as a society.

I hope this book helped you realize the impact that playing team sports had in your life. I also hope you realize the potential impact it could have on those who have not yet gotten in the game or had the experience to play. You have so much to look forward to. When I first pushed to get in the game of street ball with the boys so many years ago, I never knew that I was just beginning to have team play experiences that would shape my life. Look at me now. I am still playing and associating those skills in both my personal and professional life. Just as I had no idea how great the possibilities were, I want to suggest that you too have only just begun to realize how life-changing team play can be. *You Can Play!*

APPENDIX: A
Survey Summary

To get as many women as possible to experience the joy and rewards of playing team sports, there needs to be many opportunities from which to choose. My vision is to inspire and initiate programs throughout the country where women can play. This program, called "Women Who Play," could be incorporated within different national organizations, such as the National Parks and Recreation. For more information, check out our web site: **www.youcanplay.org**

Prior to the creation of this book, I distributed a survey titled *Women and Team Play*. I received over 2,029 surveys from women 17-to-80 years of age. The survey consisted of 36 questions based on how team play impacted a woman's life. Of the respondents, 26% or 430 women were interested in sharing their story in how playing team sports impacted their life, personally and professionally. As a result, I was able to interview and capture a handful of the stories to share in the book. My goal is to reach out to all of the women interested in sharing their personal stories about how team sports translated into success in different aspects of their life and share these stories with others.

The top life lessons learned from playing team sports:

- 84% learned that playing together builds camaraderie

- 84% learned to work together to achieve a common goal

- 82% learned that playing sports is fun

- 78% learned to be a good team member

- 75% learned that winning takes practice

- 74% learned that sports help women build self-confidence

- 73% learned the importance of communication

Seventy-seven percent of the respondents were currently on a team in their professional or personal lives. The top skills and lessons learned from team play, that 1,137 women found to be useful in their work and personal life, will be shared on the web site: **www.youcanplay.org**

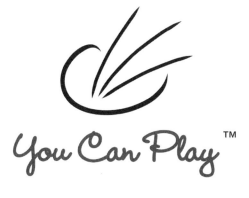

You Can Play™

Take time to Play

Experience Teamwork

Practice and Perfect Your Skills

Push Beyond your Limits

Take Risks

Celebrate Your Successes

Remember......

You Can Play

APPENDIX: B
Playbook Summary

CHAPTER 1
As you consider getting into the game, keep these tips in mind:

1. **Make play one of your top five priorities.**
   I challenge you to play something new and different that you have always wanted to try. Start a neighborhood volleyball game one night a week or sign up for a recreational soccer league. If there were a whiffle ball or kickball league, would you play? The experience ahead of you is so amazing that you will ask yourself, "Why have I been waiting so long to sign up and play?"

2. **Overcome your barriers.**
   The only thing stopping you is – you. Is the fear of the unknown standing in your way? You need a simple strategy to break down your barriers:

   - Turn loose any negative experiences from the past.

   - Set your mind on building new, positive experiences.

- Identify a sport or activity that you know you will enjoy and can be successful in trying. Just try it.

- Find others who will encourage you to try something new. Make a commitment to enjoy the experience together.

- If you are unable to find something that fits your interests, start something yourself. Invite others to join you in your game, right where you need it to be.

3. **Let play evolve to fit your life changes, and always play with others.**
   Play not only looks different for each of us as individuals, but our definition of play will also evolve and change during our lifetime. Each person needs to define play for herself. Whatever it looks like to you, play each day and enjoy it!

CHAPTER 2
As you focus on your teamwork skills, keep these tips in mind:

1. **Evaluate your skills.**
   Think about the skills you bring to a team. Whether you are a spectator, supporter, player, captain or coach, you can impact others in a positive way.

2. **Remember that teamwork takes practice.**
   Just like any other skill, it takes practice and dedication to become a successful team member. Work on soft skills such as reflective listening, openness to new ideas, strong work ethic and dedication. These will pay enormous dividends over time.

3. **Recognize your own successes.**
   Find the confidence it takes to step out in an attempt to influence others.

CHAPTER 3
As you challenge your personal limits, keep these tips in mind:

1. **Identify your goal.**
   Think about additional activities you would like to experience and enjoy.

2. **Assess your starting point.**
   Seek out an opportunity to join a team, then develop and learn at a pace that challenges you, while building your confidence.

3. **Get out there and get in the game.**
   Set aside concerns or inhibitions you have about the contribution you may make to a team and focus on the potential you have as an individual.

4. **Constantly set a new finish line for yourself.**
   Once you reach your goal, reshape it. Remember, no one is in your way but yourself. Don't settle for the status quo.

CHAPTER 4
As you consider taking new risks, keep these tips in mind:

1. **Risk = Opportunity.**
   What makes every risk worth taking is the opportunity that lies on the other side. Those who can quickly acknowledge a challenge that is presented with this mindset will move on to reap greater rewards in a more timely fashion. Remember the old saying, "There are two ways to climb an oak tree. You can climb it or you can sit on an acorn and wait for it to grow." Need I say more?

2. **Start small.**
   Begin building your confidence by extending beyond your comfort zone in situations you perceive as less risky. Make decisions that impact mostly yourself and are seen only by a small group and with little or no financial implications. Your success will prepare you for the next opportunity.

3. **Know yourself.**
   Be aware of your risk tolerance. The goal is to stretch your boundaries but not too far outside your confidence zone. Working within your tolerated level of risk will allow you to function at your best and build your confidence to take on the larger risks.

4. **Engage others.**
   Identify teams that are supportive of your proposed risk. At lower levels of risk, these people may not be affected much by your success or rewards. As the level of your chosen risks grows, the level of engagement by your team members will expand as well. They may invest time, money and talent in your cause and they will reap the rewards of your success as well as the success of the team.

5. **Be prepared.**
   Before you commit, confirm that you have the resources necessary to be successful. This includes your personal skills, the most current and accurate information surrounding the risk, support from others and financial resources.

6. **Check your mindset.**
   Focus appropriately on the opportunities and rewards, while keeping the risk in perspective. Are you confident that you will be successful in reaching your goals? Are you ready to engage others in whatever level of support you need? Are you prepared to share the rewards with your team?

7. **Decide and act.**
   Make decisions and act with confidence to move forward with your challenges. Once you have identified your interest or passion, assess the opportunity and engage others at the right level. Don't look back.

8. **Be flexible and realistic.**
   Don't be afraid to modify your plan as you uncover new information. We can all appreciate when life deals us the opportunity to run

straight up the middle and score. In reality, you will need to bob and weave with some fancy footwork to win. Not only might the process look different, but success also does not always look the same as you once envisioned. This could mark the beginning of new experiences.

CHAPTER 5

Here are a few things to keep in mind when considering which teams to join:

1. **Play with others.**
   Find your preferred interest in play or your suppressed desire with play. Playing and teams go hand-in-hand.

2. **Engage others.**
   Life is about relating to and being with people.

3. **Develop relationship skills.**
   Building relationships is the foundation for life.

4. **Change is inevitable.**
   Adaptation is the course for success.

5. **Seek others and form teams.**
   Our relationships grow through networking.

CHAPTER 6

Here are a few additional thoughts to keep in mind when considering the value of practicing with a team:

1. **Start today.**
   Start today. Only you can make it happen for yourself. You have so much to gain from this new experience. If you believe it is important to live for today and live out each moment to its fullest, then you will embrace this opportunity to play for

so many reasons.

2. **You are never too old to learn.**

   When you stop learning, you stop living. Allow yourself a few minutes each day visualizing what it would look like to play something that you have always wanted to. What does it feel like? What emotions did you display? With whom did you share it? What feeling did it leave you with? After experiencing this mental exercise for a period of time, try it on for size and make it a reality. Keep practicing, so you will reap the joy of feeling good about yourself and working through new situation.

3. **It takes a community.**

   Surround yourself with others with whom you have fun and enjoy spending time. Think about the community you can build for yourself. Who will you invite to be part of this experience? Start today and make a list of those close friends and family members with whom you wish to play.

CHAPTER 7
Here are a few things to keep in mind as you enhance your ability to think on your feet:

1. **Let go of old paradigms.**

   Tentativeness based on past experience or others' expectations can make it difficult to make decisions. When you do take the lead, be mentally prepared to think and act decisively in that team leadership position. Remember, your opinion as a team member matters – so express it.

2. **Be accountable.**

   Whether the decision you make leads to the perfect outcome or some portion thereof, be confident that you made the best decision you could given what you knew at the time. Be accountable to your team members. There are always things to be learned. If the decision was yours, own it!

3. **Trust yourself.**

   Make a decision, go with it, and see what happens. You will never know your capabilities unless you go with your gut feelings when the opportunity presents itself.

4. **Know your role.**

   If you want a safe place to ask questions and make on-the-spot decisions, a team-focused culture must be in place. This approach will ensure a friendly environment to ask questions while in pursuit of making informed decisions. Once you have found the right team, let it be known that you are ready and willing to think on your feet and act decisively on their behalf – and that you are ready to be accountable.

5. **Seize the opportunity.**

   On any team, some are comfortable thinking on their feet. Others, meanwhile, have great ideas but aren't ready to step up to the plate. It feels good to take the lead; act decisively and enjoy success. Practice seizing small opportunities as a first step.

CHAPTER 8

Keep these things in mind as you work to leverage and learn from your mistakes:

1. **We all make mistakes.**

   Don't try to be a perfectionist. Accept the fact that you will make mistakes.

2. **Mistakes are opportunities to learn.**

   You will make smarter mistakes in the future.

3. **Share your mistakes.**

   Go to the people who need to know and discuss what happened.

4. **Assess the lessons learned.**
   Take notes on the entire experience and make sure you make the most of it.

5. **Engage others who you respect that can influence your learning curve.**
   Create your own team huddle.

6. **Make a plan.**
   Find ways you can stay clear of making the same mistakes.

CHAPTER 9
Here are a few things to keep in mind when learning to be competitive:

1. **Give yourself permission to compete.**
   Pay attention to what comes to mind when you think about competing. Be mindful of your feelings, both positive and negative. Take a moment to shift any negative perceptions so you can begin to look at competition as a good thing.

2. **Do the mental preparation.**
   Imagine how you would feel. Envision the outcome. Repeat the behavior so it sticks and begins to feel like a part of who you are.

3. **Learn to win as a team.**
   Recall the role you have played in the past on a winning team. Think about the gifts that you brought to the team that helped them win. Remember the experience and the feeling of victory.

4. **Translate a winning attitude into individual victories.**
   Think about how your own winning profile can translate into other parts of your life.

5. **Recognize the small victories.**
   There are small victories that we experience every day, yet we often fail to recognize them. Write down the next stepping stones toward

your larger goal. When you accomplish one of these steps of success, recognize it, celebrate it and tally the win.

6. **Learn to enjoy the feeling of the win.**
Visualize how you feel, illustrating the picture in your memory. Draw on it as you prepare to compete in individual or team sports. The positive energy from winning should never be overlooked. Always celebrate it and feed off of it for the future.

7. **Understand that the experience will be greater than you can imagine.**
Trust in the positive results and allow yourself permission to keep the feeling alive. Would you feel differently if you won?

CHAPTER 10
Here are some things to keep in mind when planning to celebrate success:

1. **Picture the win before you even get started.**
Mental preparation is probably a greater contributor to success than physical preparation. Even the most talented fall short of victory if they do not have the right attitude and mindset to win.

2. **Recognize and celebrate the small wins.**
Don't underestimate the reward and motivation that comes from celebrating small victories on your way to the bigger win.

3. **Define victory based on your personal goals.**
Refrain from worrying about what others think. Remember that every small victory builds your confidence and brings you closer to the larger victory.

4. **Practice rules of common courtesy in your approach to celebrating.**
A simple set of rules will go a long way toward making you feel comfortable with celebrating publicly and reinforcing this life skill.

5. **Recognize all victories.**

   Treat each and every little win like it is the first and the last. Take notice of the little or unexpected victories. Celebration takes practice and will become a habit when you get it right.

6. **Encourage others to celebrate their victories.**

ABOUT
BRENDA LOUBE, M.S.

Brenda Loube has devoted her life to fitness, health promotion, disease prevention and sports As a young girl, Brenda got into any game she could, with family, friends or at school. During high school, she received varsity letters in basketball, volleyball, field hockey and softball. In college, she played competitive softball and tennis. As an adult, Brenda became a nationally ranked racquetball player, leading to many championships and her 1993 induction into the Jewish Sports Hall of Fame.

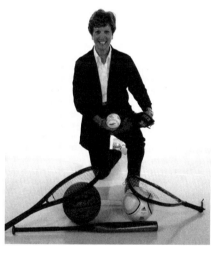

She taught physical education at the middle-school level, as well as coached a number of teams at the high-school and collegiate level. Brenda then became intrigued with cardiac rehabilitation and pursued her master's degree. She later served as a graduate assistant and ultimately founded Georgetown University Hospital's inpatient and outpatient cardiac rehabilitation program.

After working as the program director for multiple commercial health clubs, Brenda co-founded Corporate Fitness Works in 1988. Today, she serves as principal and co-founder for the company, which provides fitness-center planning, facility management and fitness and wellness consulting services for corporations, government agencies and residential and retirement communities. The company's mission is to set the standard for creating cultures that encourage individual and corporate well-being.

Brenda has been active in a wide range of professional and non-profit organizations, including Women Presidents' Organization; American College of Sports Medicine; Association for Worksite Health Promotion; Wellness Councils of America; the American Alliance for Health, Physical Education, Recreation and Dance; and the International Council on Active Aging. In 2000, she was appointed to the Maryland Governor's Council on Physical Fitness, where she has served as chairperson since 2004. Brenda is currently a member of the board of directors for the International Association for Worksite Health Promotion and the National Association for Health and Fitness, and is a member of the advisory board for the International Council on Active Aging.

Brenda has been recognized with numerous business and leadership awards including:

- National "Exemplary Health and Fitness Leadership Award" from the National Association for Health and Fitness

- "The President's Council on Physical Fitness and Sports Community Leadership Award"

- "The Dean's Award for the Department of Health Professions" from Towson University

- "WBENC Business Star Award" from the Women's Business Enterprise National Council

- "William G. Anderson Award" from The American Alliance for Health, Physical Education, Recreation and Dance

- "Outstanding Women Business Enterprises Award" from the Women Presidents' Educational Organization

- "Health Educator of the Year Award in the Worksite Category" from The American Alliance for Health, Physical Education, Recreation and Dance

Being a business owner has been Brenda's vehicle for living out her dreams. She learned early in her career that we really can prevent heart disease and other lifestyle-related illnesses. She has had the opportunity for the past 36 years to increase awareness and education and to develop strategies to assist her clients' employees and residents in disease prevention through lifestyle management habits. Her continued and primary motivation to grow her business is to provide new employment opportunities and professional growth for those in the fields of physical education, exercise science, health promotion and other related areas who want to spread her message of fitness and wellness to the general population. Brenda's true passion is to coach her team to assist its members in improving quality of life. She feels everyone deserves to be healthy and to reach their optimal health and well-being.

Brenda earned a bachelor's degree in physical education from Towson University and her master's degree in physical education with an emphasis in cardiac rehabilitation from the University of Wisconsin – LaCrosse.

CORPORATE FITNESS WORKS
COMPANY OVERVIEW

Corporate Fitness Works is a certified woman-owned company that has been offering comprehensive fitness solutions to corporations, government agencies and residential communities throughout the nation since 1988. Founded by two women with one vision, Corporate Fitness Works has extended project-management experience to successfully conceptualize, develop and manage fitness centers ranging from 1,000 to 70,000 square feet for populations from 500 to 14,000 individuals.

Corporate Fitness Works treats each client relationship as a partnership, which is evident through the complete alignment and integration of services into an organization's own culture. Working with clients on an individual basis, Corporate Fitness Works is able to develop, equip and manage the best facilities that provide targeted programs and services in order to achieve specific goals and objectives. Proven operational and programming systems are aligned with clients' stated objectives for the facility and program, which in turn are implemented by Corporate Fitness Works' degreed professionals. From the on-site fitness and wellness teams to executive leaders, all Corporate Fitness Works team members have a deeply rooted conviction for enhancing the health and well-being of client populations. Combined with a passion for service excellence, this translates to a commitment for quality service delivery, accountability and consistent performance. These best practices yield exceptional customer satisfaction ratings of consistently over 98% and create a culture of happier, healthier and more productive individuals. Our commitment is to set the standard for creating well cultures that encourage individual and overall well-being. To learn more, explore **www.corporatefitnessworks.com**.

Invite Brenda to Speak to Your Group

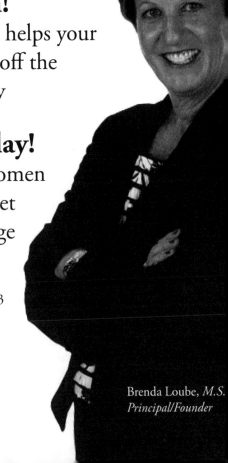

You Can Play!
Inspiring presentations from the book, tailored to your group

To Your Health!
Motivational coach helps your corporate team get off the bench and into play

Women Can Play!
Why don't more women play team sports? Let other women change your life this year

Phone: 301-417-9697 ext 1113
Fax: 301-417-0651

BrendaSpeaks@YouCanPlay.org
www.YouCanPlay.org

Brenda Loube, *M.S.*
Principal/Founder